The Ultimate Cooking Companion *for* At-Home Caregivers

Mary Ellen Capron, MS, RD
Elana Zucker, RN, MSN

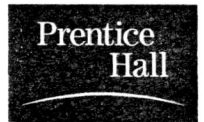

Upper Saddle River, New Jersey 07458

Library of Congress Cataloging-in-Publication Data

Capron, Mary Ellen.
  The ultimate cooking companion for at-home caregivers/by Mary Ellen Capron, Elana Zucker.
    p. cm.
  ISBN 0-13-019440-9 (alk. paper)
  1. Cookery for the sick. 2. Home health aides. I. Zucker, Elana D., (date)-II. Title.
  RM219. C26 2003
  613.2—dc21   2002022477

Publisher: Julie Levin Alexander
Assistant to Publisher: Regina Bruno
Executive Editor: Maura Connor
Acquisitions Editor: Barbara Krawiec
Editorial Assistant: Sheba Jalaluddin
Director of Manufacturing and Production: Bruce Johnson
Managing Production Editor: Patrick Walsh
Production Liaison: Mary C. Treacy
Production Editor: Linda Begley, Rainbow Graphics
Manufacturing Manager: Ilene Sanford
Manufacturing Buyer: Pat Brown
Design Director: Cheryl Asherman
Senior Design Coordinator: Maria Guglielmo Walsh
Interior Design: Wanda España
Senior Marketing Manager: Nicole Benson
Marketing Coordinator: Janet Ryerson
Product Information Manager: Rachele Strober
Composition: Rainbow Graphics
Cover Photo: Paul Poplis/Foodpix
Cover Printer: Phoenix Color Corporation
Printing and Binding: RR Donnelley, Harrisonburg, VA

Pearson Education LTD.
Pearson Education Australia PTY, Limited
Pearson Education Singapore, Pte. Ltd
Pearson Education North Asia Ltd
Pearson Education Canada, Ltd.
Pearson Educación de Mexico, S.A. de C.V.
Pearson Education–Japan
Pearson Education Malaysia, Pte. Ltd
Pearson Education, Upper Saddle River, New Jersey

NOTICE
The procedures described in the textbook are based on consultation with nursing assistant authorities. The author and publisher have taken care to make certain that these procedures reflect currently accepted clinical practice; however, they cannot be considered absolute recommendations.

The material in this textbook contains the most current information available at the time of publication. However, federal, state, and local guidelines concerning clinical practices, including, without limitation, those governing infection control and universal precautions, change rapidly. The reader should note, therefore, that new regulations may require changes in some procedures.

It is the responsibility of the reader to familiarize himself or herself with the policies set by federal, state, and local agencies, as well as the supplements written to accompany it, disclaim any liability, loss, or risk resulting directly or indirectly from the suggested procedures and theory, from any undetected errors, or from the reader's misunderstanding of the text. It is the reader's responsibility to stay informed of any new changes or recommendations made by any federal, state, and local agency as well as by his or her employing health care institution or agency.

Copyright © 2003 by Prentice-Hall, Inc., Upper Saddle River, New Jersey 07458. All rights reserved. Printed in the United States of America. This publication is protected by Copyright and permission should be obtained from the publisher prior to any prohibited reproduction, storage in a retrieval system, or transmission in any form or by any means, electronic, mechanical, photocopying, recording, or likewise. For information regarding permission(s), write to: Rights and Permissions Department.

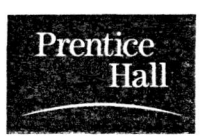

10 9 8 7 6 5 4 3 2 1
ISBN 0-13-019440-9

Contents

PREFACE IX

GENERAL RECIPE INTRODUCTION XI

ABOUT THE AUTHORS XIII

1 **BASIC NUTRITION** 1
Nutrients 1
The Food Pyramid 6
The Dietary Guidelines 9
Vegetarians 11
Your Role as a Homemaker/Home Health Aide 11

2 **FOOD SUPPLEMENTS, HERBAL SUPPLEMENTS, VITAMINS** 13
Supporting a Client Taking Supplements 14
Herbal Preparations and Antioxidants 15
Vitamins and Minerals 16
Your Role as a Homemaker/Home Health Aide 18

3 **FEEDING A CLIENT** 21
Assisting a Client with Feeding 22
Planning to Feed a Client 22
Basic Considerations 23
Physical Limitations 23
Safety Factors 24
Feeding Children 25
Physical Abilities of Children 29
Cleaning Up 29
Your Role as a Homemaker/Home Health Aide 30

4 **CULTURAL ASPECTS OF FOOD** 31
Influences on Food Choices 31
How We Eat 33
Changing What We Eat 34
Changing Is Difficult 34
Your Role as a Homemaker/Home Health Aide 34

iii

5 Kitchen Staples 37
Determining the Staples for Your Client 38
Your Role as a Homemaker/Home Health Aide 41

6 Shopping for Food and Reading the Food Label 43
Before You Get to the Store 43
At the Store 44
Unit Pricing 45
Reading a Food Label 45
Stretching the Food Dollar 46
When You Return Home 47
Your Role as a Homemaker/Home Health Aide 47

7 Storage and Handling of Food 49
Handling Foods Safely 50
Using the Refrigerator Safely 50
Using the Freezer Safely 53
Using Microwave Ovens Safely 53
Defrosting Foods 54
Pantry Storage 54
Dating of Food Products 55
Tips for Cooking Safely 55
Your Role as a Homemaker/Home Health Aide 56

8 Sodium-Restricted Diet 59
Why the Body Needs Sodium 59
Sodium Levels in the Body 60
Maintaining a Sodium-Restricted Diet 60
The Impact of a Sodium-Restricted Diet 61
Helpful Hints 61
Using Herbs and Spices 63
Your Role as a Homemaker/Home Health Aide 63

9 Fat- and Cholesterol-Restricted Diets 65
Fats 66
Cholesterol 67
Changing Cooking Habits 69
Olestra 69
Your Role as a Homemaker/Home Health Aide 70

10 Diabetic Diets 71
Who Is at Risk for Diabetes? 71
Signs and Symptoms of Diabetes Mellitus 72

The Importance of Maintaining a Diabetic Diet 73
Guidelines to Maintaining a Diabetic Diet 73
Eating in a Restaurant 74
Signs and Symptoms of Diabetic Coma 74
Signs and Symptoms of Insulin Shock 75
Your Role as a Homemaker/Home Health Aide 75

11 ADDITIONAL DIETARY CONSIDERATIONS AND MODIFICATIONS 77
Dietary Fiber 77
Adding Fiber to a Diet 79
Low-Residue or Low-Fiber Diet 79
Clear Liquid Diet 79
Full Liquid Diet 80
Soft Diet 81
Mechanical Soft Diet 81
Pureed Diet 81
Dysphagia Diets 82
Low-Lactose or Lactose-Free Diet 82
Your Role as a Homemaker/Home Health Aide 83

12 FOOD AND DRUG INTERACTIONS 85
How Food and Drug Interactions Occur 86
Drugs and the Elderly 86
Balancing Drug Administration with Meals 87
The Five Rights of Medication Administration 87
Medication Labels 88
Medication Storage 88
Herbal Supplements 89
General Guidelines of Common Food
  and Drug Interactions 89
Drugs and Alcohol 92
Your Role as a Homemaker/Home Health Aide 93

13 FEEDING DIFFICULTIES AND ALTERNATIVES 95
Loss of Appetite 95
Bloating/Edema 96
Gas 97
Sore Mouth or Throat 97
Nausea/Vomiting 98
Constipation 99
Diarrhea 99
Enteral Nutrition 100
Total Parenteral Nutrition 101
Your Role as a Homemaker/Home Health Aide 101

Contents v

14 Recipes for Soup 103
   Bean Soup   105
   Chicken Broth   106
   Lentil Soup   107
   Minestrone   108
   Split Pea Soup   109
   Tomato Soup   110
   Turkey Vegetable Soup   111
   Vegetable Soup   112

15 Recipes for Entrées: Beef, Lamb, Pork, Poultry, Fish, and Meatless 113
   Beef Stew (quick)   115
   Chili   116
   Meatloaf   117
   Pepper Steak   118
   Pot Roast   119
   Sloppy Joes   120
   Braised Lamb Shanks   122
   Lamb Chops   123
   Pork Medallions   125
   Pork Stir-Fry   126
   Boneless Chicken Breast Sautéed   129
   Chicken Cutlets Breaded   130
   Chicken Fricassee   131
   Chicken, Grilled   132
   Chicken, Marinated   133
   Chicken Parmigiana   134
   Chicken/Turkey Sausage with Onions,
      Peppers, and Mushrooms   135
   Turkey Burgers   136
   Baked Fish   138
   Creole Fish   139
   Pan-Fried Fish   140
   Eggplant Parmigiana (low fat)   142
   Macaroni and Cheese   143
   Pasta Primavera   144
   Quick Tomato Sauce   145
   Stuffed Shells   146

16 Recipes for Vegetables 147
   Baked Acorn Squash   149
   Broccoli, Steamed   150
   Carrots (basic)   151
   Grated Zucchini   152
   Green Beans Sauté   153

Vegetables, Canned   154
Vegetables, Frozen   155

17 Recipes for Rice, Potato, and Pasta   157
Brown Rice   159
Fried Rice Chinese Style   160
Rice and Beans   161
Rice Indian Style   162
Rice Mexican Style   163
Rice Pilaf   164
Rice with Lentils   165
Baked Potato (oven and microwave)   166
Boiled Potato   167
Home Fried Potatoes   168
Mashed Potatoes   169
Potato Croquettes   170
Rosemary Garlic Sweet Potatoes   171
Roasted Potatoes   172
Pasta with Beans   173
Pasta with Butter   174
Pasta with Garlic and Oil   175
Pasta with Herbs and Cheese   176
Pasta with Quick Tomato Sauce   177
Barley with Mushrooms   178
Grits Casserole   179
Quinoa   180
Tabbouleh   181

18 Recipes for Fruit   183
Baked Apples   185
Broiled Grapefruit   186
Cooked Fruit Compote   187
Fruit Cubes   188
Glazed Bananas   189
Nectarine and Cantaloupe Smoothie   190
Pureed Fruit with Whipped Topping   191

19 Recipes for Eggs and Cheese   193
Blintzes   195
Cheese Filling for Blintzes   196
Cheese Quesadillas   197
Egg Salad   198
French Toast   199
Frittata   200
Omelet   201
Quiche   202
Strata   203

20 Recipes for Salad   205
Carrot and Raisin Salad   207
Chef's Salad   208
Cole Slaw   209
Potato Salad   210
Rice and Vegetable Salad   211
Spinach Salad   212
Three-Bean Salad   213
Tuna Fish Salad   214
Vegetable Salad   215
Balsamic Vinaigrette   216
Basic Lemon Dressing   217
Blue Cheese Dressing   218
Lemon Garlic Mayonnaise   219

21 Recipes for Sandwiches   221
English Muffin Pizza   224
Grilled Cheese   225
Roasted Vegetable Sandwich   226
Turkey and Cheese Roll-Up   227

22 Recipes for Beverages   229
Blended Banana   231
Café au Lait   232
Creamsicle   233
Enriched Iced Coffee   234
Fruit Freeze   235
Hot Apple Cider   236
Strawberry Milk Smoothie   237
Vanilla Milkshake   238
Yogurt Smoothie   239

23 Recipes for Snacks   241
Apple Crisp   242
Blueberry Muffins   243
Bran Muffins   244
Corn Bread   245
Fritters   246
Fruity Spread for Graham Crackers   247
Raisin Oatmeal Bars   248
Rice Pudding   249

Appendix   251

Glossary   261

Index   265

Preface

A multidisciplinary team of practicing home care, nutrition, and education professionals has compiled *The Ultimate Cooking Companion for At-Home Caregivers*. It is well known that food and the associated activities are meaningful to clients and contribute very positively to the health and well-being of people. This book contains information to assist the homemaker/home health aide as they plan and cook meals, assist clients and families with feeding, and model the very best nutritional-related practices. The goal is to assist the aide in establishing a nutritionally sound atmosphere so that nutrition will be maintained when the aide is no longer in the home. The book is designed to enhance the experience of eating!

Information is presented in a clear, concise manner so that it can be used both as an initial introduction to the subjects and as a quick review. The principles contained in the book contribute to the homemaker/home health aides' achieving job satisfaction in an atmosphere of safety while modeling appropriate behaviors so the client can achieve a maximum level of function.

This text is a basic offering of tested recipes, which can be expanded on and personalized for clients, as their diet preferences require. Suggestions and areas appropriate for changes are indicated with each recipe. This unique feature allows the homemaker/home health aide to individualize care for all clients regardless of their dietary requirements.

KEY FEATURES

- Each recipe is *culturally sensitive* to enable the user to adapt it when needed.
- The text is *age sensitive* so that the user will be able to adapt the recipes for children, the elderly, and physically impaired of all ages.
- The *role of the homemaker/home health aide* as caregiver, team member, and role model is presented in clear and concise language.
- *New words* are printed in boldface within the text. The glossary on pages 261–264 presents all the words in one place for reference.

CHAPTER HIGHLIGHTS

- The *Introduction* to each chapter presents an overview of the chapter content. It sets the stage for the material to follow by summarizing the roles of the homemaker/home health aide, the client, and the material.

- *Subject headings* enhance the ability of the aide in identifying the material so that the aid upon initial study and later when you use the text as a reference.
- *Points to remember* summarize the chapter content and identify the most salient points of the preceding material. They also provide points of discussion in a classroom setting.
- *Recipe format* provides, on one page, *all* pertinent information relating to the preparation of the dish, including preparation time, basic preparation steps, suggestions for changes associated with age, physical limitations, cultural requirements, and calorie and fat content.

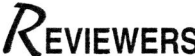REVIEWERS

Mary Jo Clark
Nurse Consultant

Ann M. Larson, RN, PhN, BS
Instructor
Minneapolis Community and Technical College
Minneapolis, MN

General Recipe Introduction

Recipes are very personal possessions. They reflect our personal taste, our culture, and our family transitions. Recipes are handed down from generation to generation as personal possessions and reminders of favorite people or experiences. They can change over time or remain the same as we choose. Your clients will also have personal favorite recipes. As you plan meals, shop, and cook for your clients, respect their preferences. These preferences are important to them and contribute to their enjoyment of the food and the eating experience.

The recipes in this book are designed to be used as a basic simple guideline for the dish. The recipes can be changed and altered to taste and experience. There are many suggestions for changes that would be appropriate. Your client may have others. You may have others. Remember that some people do not like change, so discuss with your client before you make changes in recipes. Remember that some people have specific limitations on foods that cannot be consumed due to medical conditions.

The recipes in this book were constructed carefully and thoughtfully and provide several areas for individualization.

- The recipes include prep time and cooking time. Use these times as a guide.
- Salt and pepper is an individual preference. Therefore, it has intentionally been omitted from all recipes and not included in the ***analysis.*** You are reminded to discuss the addition of salt and pepper with your client. Refer to Table C for this information.
- All spices are assumed to be dried in the analysis, but fresh can be used.
- If you are using a prepared seasoning, read the label to determine if salt is one of the ingredients.
- Words listed in substitutions that are in ***italics and bold*** indicate that this will change the nutrient content for one or more nutrients and Table C should be referred to for changes in nutrient content.
- If using a microwave, cover the food with wax paper or plastic wrap before cooking it. Baking potatoes is the exception. Discuss with the client the usual timing in his or her microwave. Not all are the same.
- All ovens and stoves are different. When times are present in the recipe, they are guidelines. You will have to adjust the time to your cooking equipment.
- You may cook half a recipe, but each serving will still have the same analysis as when you cook the whole recipe.

- You may also notice that the **yield** may be different than indicated in the book. Yields often differ depending on the cooking temperature and the cooking method. The yields are also guides and useful to determine serving size, but should not be taken as an absolute.
- If you refrigerate or freeze food, the seasoning often has to be readjusted after the food has thawed.
- When pureeing food it may be necessary to add liquid and/or a thickening agent to achieve the desired consistency of the food.
- To puree or mash food you may use either a fork, a food mill, a strainer, or a blender.
- Food is always pureed after the cooking process is completed.
- Check sell date. Never buy a package past the sell date.
- If you open the package and it does not have a fresh smell, do not eat it!

About the Authors

Mary Ellen Capron, MS, RD

Mary Ellen Capron, MS, RD, has over 20 years' experience working in the health care environment. She received her master's degree in Nutrition from the University of Bridgeport and her undergraduate degree from the College of Saint Elizabeth in Morristown, New Jersey. She has worked with all age groups in acute, chronic, and short- and long-term facilities. In these facilities, she has worked as a staff person and as an administrator. At Overlook Hospital in Summit, New Jersey, she held various positions from staff dietitian to the Clinical Nutrition Manager. In this capacity, she was instrumental in formulating the diets of over 500 patients a day and of overseeing the preparation of the food. Ms. Capron was a member of various state bodies that formulated regulations for all in-patient facilities within New Jersey. As a member of the health care team, she was often called on to teach students and graduate personnel. She has worked as a nutrition consultant for several physician groups and enjoys educating the community on eating practices.

Elana D. Zucker, RN, MSN

Elana Zucker, RN, MSN, has been an active contributor to the nursing and home health care profession for 37 years. As a graduate nurse, she worked in the community in Washington D.C., New York, and New Jersey. She has helped author both federal and state legislation. She has taught at Fairleigh Dickinson University in the graduate nurse program and has been a speaker on both the state and federal level. In her capacity as administrator of a federal grant to The Home Health Agency of New Jersey to train homemakers/home health aides in New Jersey, she was the guiding force in training thousands of aides to meet the growing need for this pivotal member of the health team. In this capacity she was instrumental, establishing systems to regulate the curriculum and monitoring the credentialing of the students. Ms. Zucker has held positions at Overlook Hospital, New Jersey, as the Director of Community Health, Director of Nursing, and Chief Nursing Officer. She now focuses her energies on consulting, being an expert witness, writing, and volunteer work for a local agency that provides services to families so that their elderly adult members may remain at home.

CHAPTER 1

Basic Nutrition

Introduction

*In this chapter, you will become familiar with the food pyramid so that you will be able to plan **nutritious** meals. You will also learn about the need for each **nutrient** and the most common foods, which can supply them. Your role in helping clients meet their dietary requirements will be discussed also.*

Good nutrition is important throughout the **life cycle** regardless of age or medical condition. Food gives the body energy to carry out the day's activities and is necessary to rebuild body tissue. Eating is also a social activity. It is associated with cultural practices and family and personal preferences. In some homes, it is the time when family members come together. In some homes, everyone eats separately. In some homes, the women eat separately from the men. In some homes, the children do not eat with the adults except on special occasions. Each home is different. Do not assume that each family is the same. You will be asked to respect the practices in the home and help the family with their nutrition so that it is comfortable to them.

NUTRIENTS

Nutrients are substances that our bodies need to repair, maintain, and grow new cells. Nutrients are supplied from the food we eat. Each nutrient comes from many sources. For proper bodily function it is necessary that a balance be kept among all nutrients—not too much of one or the other.

It does not matter from which food the nutrient comes as long as it is in sufficient supply. When people are unable to get the proper amount of a nutrient from their food due to disease, physical disability, or preference, they may take **supplements** to provide one or more identified nutrients. Supplements must be prescribed by a **health care professional** and taken into account when a client's complete nutritional status is reviewed. Be sure to discuss the need for supplements with your supervisor before you assist the client with taking them.

Three Main Nutrients—Carbohydrates, Proteins, and Fats

Carbohydrates carry nutrients in foods throughout the body. Carbohydrate is the main source of energy for all activities. Think of carbohydrates as fuel for the body. Carbohydrates can be further broken down into **complex** and **simple.** Complex carbohydrates—those in the base of the pyramid—include starch and fiber. During digestion, all carbohydrates are broken down to sugar except fiber. Sugars and starches occur naturally in many foods. Carbohydrate supplies 4 calories per gram. Simple sugars are located in the tip of the pyramid, not the base. These include foods like soda, candy, and cakes and are often referred to as "empty calories" because they have little if any nutritional value. When carbohydrate is not available, the body starts to use other nutrient sources for energy, causing an imbalance in the body. For example, if carbohydrates are not available for energy, the body might use its store of protein. When protein is used for energy, it is not available for muscle and tissue repair.

Proteins form an important part of **enzymes, hormones,** and **body fluids.** They are known as the building blocks, or **essential amino acids** because they build and maintain all body tissues. Proteins or amino acids help build blood and form **antibodies** to fight infection. Protein provide 4 calories per gram. Dietary proteins are found in meats, fish, poultry, eggs, milk products, and some vegetable products like soybeans, legumes, and beans. Essential amino acids must be obtained from food sources as they are not **synthesized** in the body. Inadequate intake of any essential amino acids will cause nutritional imbalance resulting in weight loss, impaired growth in infants and children, and many other symptoms.

Fat adds variety and taste to the diet and is considered a secondary source of energy. Fat supplies **essential fatty acids** that keep the skin healthy and carries and stores fat-soluble vitamins (A, D, E, and K). All fats are not the same. **Saturated fats** tend to raise blood cholesterol levels. These are the fats that are hard at room temperature. Animal products, whole milk, cheese, ice cream, and some vegetable oils like coconut and palm oil are high in saturated fats. **Cholesterol,** one type of fat, is found only in animal products. It is a soft, waxy substance. The body produces cholesterol naturally because it needs it in small amounts. All the cholesterol that is eaten is extra. Cholesterol is not the same as saturated fat. A food can be low in cholesterol but high in saturated fats. **Unsaturated fats** in the diet are beneficial to the body. They include nuts, vegetable oils, and some soft margarine products. To make some vegetable oils more versatile, they are often hydrogenated. **Hydrogenation** is a process by which some fats are hardened. These fats then act like saturated fats and need to be limited in the diet.

Calories

The combination of carbohydrate, protein, and fat all supply energy to the body in the form of **calories** to enable the body to work. Calories are needed for proper growth, development, and maintenance. The amount of calories one needs depends on many things, such as:

- Activity
- Medical conditions
- Health status

The number of calories your client should have must be discussed with your supervisor, as this forms an essential part of the framework for meal planning.

Vitamins and Micronutrients

Foods supply the body with carbohydrate, protein, fat, **vitamins,** and **minerals.** Vitamins and minerals are **micronutrients.** Micronutrients are essential to good health but are needed in small amounts. Some minerals include potassium, calcium, and iron (Figure 1.1).

Nutrient Class	Bodily Functions	Food Sources
CARBOHYDRATES 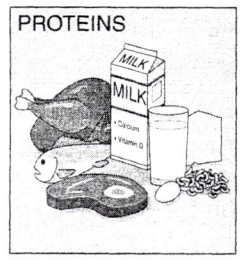	Provides work energy for body activities, and heat energy for maintenance of body temperature.	Cereal grains and their products (bread, breakfast cereals, macaroni products), potatoes, sugar, syrups, fruits, milk, vegetables, nuts.
PROTEINS	Build and renew body tissues; regulate body functions and supply energy. Complete proteins: maintain life and provide growth. Incomplete proteins: maintain life but do not provide for growth.	Complete proteins: Derived from animal foods—meat, milk, eggs, fish, cheese, poultry. Incomplete proteins: Derived from vegetable foods—soybeans, dry beans, peas, some nuts, and whole-grain products.

FIGURE 1.1 *(continued)*

Nutrient Class	Bodily Functions	Food Sources
FATS 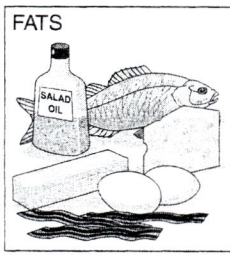	Give work energy for body activities and heat energy for maintenance of body temperature. Carrier of vitamins A and D, provide fatty acids necessary for growth and maintenance of body tissues.	Some foods are chiefly fat, such as lard, vegetable fats and oils, and butter. Many other foods contain smaller proportions of fats—nuts, meats, fish, poultry, cream, whole milk.
MINERALS Calcium 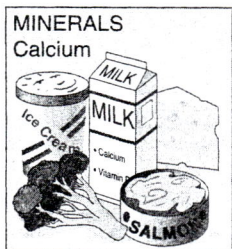	Builds and renews bones, teeth, and other tissues; regulates the activity of the muscles, heart, nerves; and controls the clotting of blood.	Milk and milk products except butter; most dark green vegetables; canned salmon. 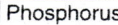 *with bones*
Phosphorus 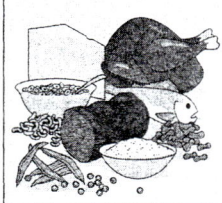	Associated with calcium in some functions needed to build and renew bones and teeth. Influences the oxidation of foods in the body cells; important in nerve tissue.	Widely distributed in foods; especially cheese, oat cereals, whole-wheat products, dry beans and peas, meat, fish, poultry, nuts.
Iron 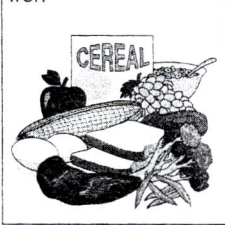	Builds and renews hemoglobin, the red pigment in blood which carries oxygen from the lungs to the cells.	Eggs, meat, especially liver and kidney; deep-yellow and dark green vegetables; potatoes, dried fruits, whole-grain products; enriched flour, bread, breakfast cereals.
Iodine 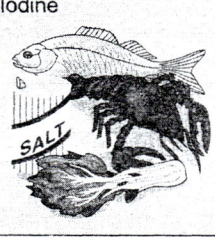	Enables the thyroid gland to perform its function of controlling the rate at which foods are oxidized in the cells.	Fish (obtained from the sea), some plant-foods grown in soils containing iodine; table salt fortified with iodine (iodized).

FIGURE 1.1 *(continued)*

Nutrient Class	Bodily Functions	Food Sources
VITAMINS A 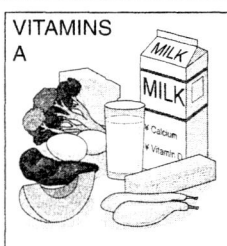	Necessary for normal functioning of the eyes, prevents night blindness. Ensures a healthy condition of the skin, hair, and mucous membranes. Maintains a state of resistance to infections of the eyes, mouth, and respiratory tract.	One form of vitamin A is yellow and one form is colorless. Apricots, cantaloupe, milk, cheese, eggs, meat organs, (especially liver and kidney), fortified margarine, butter, fish-liver oils, dark green and deep yellow vegetables.
B Complex B_1 (Thiamine) 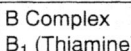 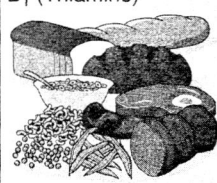	Maintains a healthy condition of the nerves. Fosters a good appetite. Helps the body cells use carbohydrates.	Whole-grain and enriched grain products; meats (especially pork, liver and kidney). Dry beans and peas.
B_2 (Riboflavin) 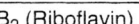 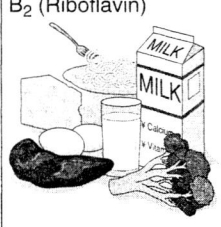	Keeps the skin, mouth, and eyes in a healthy condition. Acts with other nutrients to form enzymes and control oxidation in cells.	Milk, cheese, eggs, meat (especially liver and kidney), whole-grain and enriched grain products, dark green vegetables.
Niacin  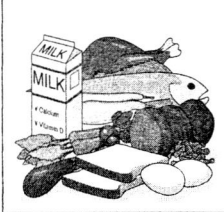	Influences the oxidation of carbohydrates and proteins in the body cells.	Liver, meat, fish, poultry, eggs, peanuts; dark green vegetables whole-grain and enriched cereal products.
B_{12} 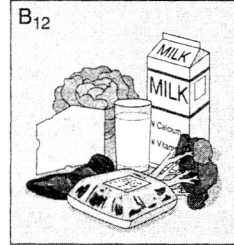	Regulates specific processes in digestion. Helps maintain normal functions of muscles, nerves, heart, blood—general body metabolism.	Liver, other organ meats, cheese, eggs, milk, leafy green vegetables.

FIGURE 1.1 *(continued)*

Nutrient Class	Bodily Functions	Food Sources
C (Ascorbic Acid) 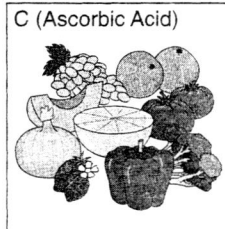	Acts as a cement between body cells, and helps them work together to carry out their special functions. Maintains a sound condition of bones, teeth, and gums. Not stored in the body.	Fresh, raw citrus fruits and vegetables—oranges, grapefruit, cantaloupe, strawberries, tomatoes, raw onions, cabbage, green and sweet red peppers, dark green vegetables.
D 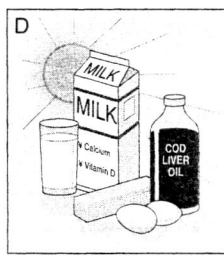	Enables the growing body to use calcium and phosphorus in a normal way to build bones and teeth.	Provided by vitamin D fortification of certain foods, such as milk and margarine. Also fish—liver oils and eggs. Sunshine is also a source of vitamin D.
WATER 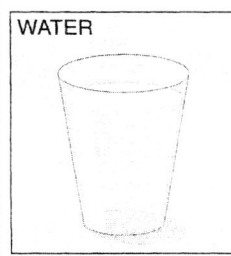	Regulates body processes. Aids in regulating body temperature. Carries nutrients to body cells and carries waste products away from them. Helps to lubricate joints. Water has no food value, although most water contains mineral elements. More immediately necessary to life than food—second only to oxygen.	Drinking water, and other beverages; all foods except those made up of a single nutrient, as sugar and some fats. Milk, milk drinks, soups, vegetables, fruit juices. Ice cream, watermelon, strawberries, lettuce, tomatoes, cereals, other dry products.

FIGURE 1.1 (continued)

THE FOOD PYRAMID

All foods have been divided into **basic food groups** and displayed in a **pyramid** shape. This was done by the U.S Department of Agriculture/U.S. Department of Health and Human Services so that everyone would have a simple guide for determining how much of each food an average adult should eat. The pyramid is a visual guide. The base is larger, and a person needs to eat more often from this part of the pyramid because the body needs more servings from the base and less as you go up.

The tip of the pyramid is small and does not even have recommended amounts of fats and sugars, as these should be consumed in **moderation** (Figure 1.2).

Calculating "One Serving"

Recommended servings are listed for each food group. A person who eats the correct number of servings from each food group will most likely get the correct amount of each nutrient the body needs for proper growth, development, and maintenance. Keep in mind that these are recommended minimums and some individuals may need more. Dietary requirements are different at different stages of life. Children need more

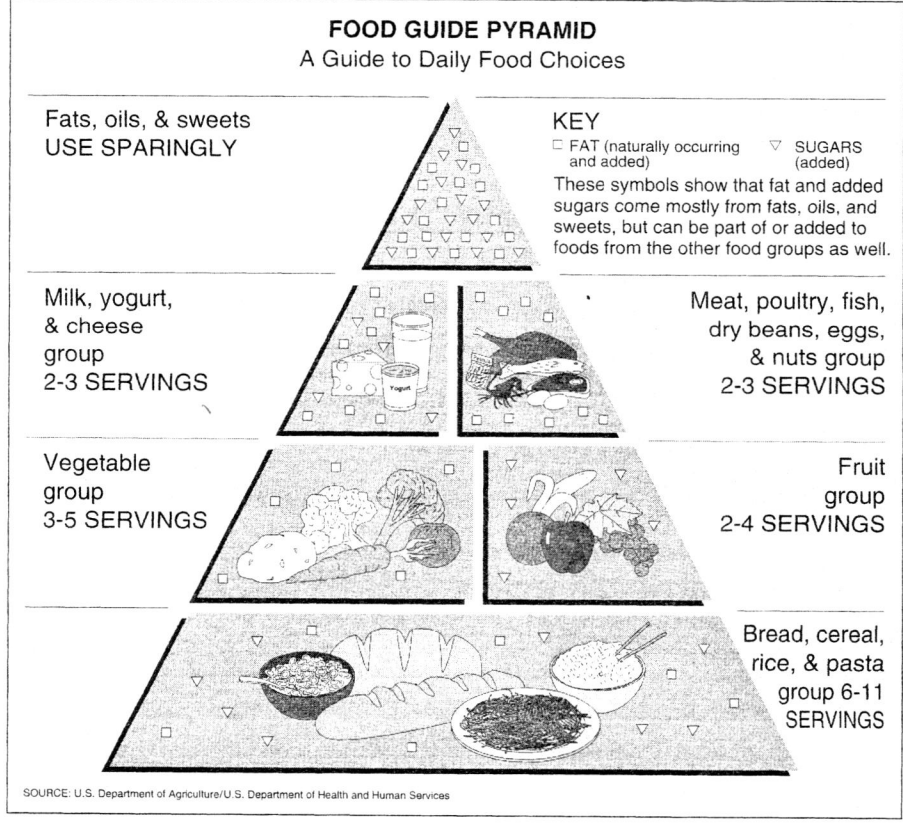

FIGURE 1.2

protein and calories than an older person needs, but older persons need more or less of other nutrients. The Food Pyramid refers to "one serving." The amount of food listed equals 1 serving from the specific food group. If you eat a larger portion, count it as more than one serving; if you eat less than listed, count it as less than a serving.

Bread, Cereal, Rice, and Pasta

1 slice of bread
1 ounce ready to eat cereal
$\frac{1}{2}$ cup cooked cereal, rice, or pasta

Fruit

1 medium apple, orange, or banana
$\frac{1}{2}$ cup canned, cooked, or chopped fruit
$\frac{3}{4}$ cup any fruit juice or $\frac{1}{2}$ cup prune juice

Vegetables

1 cup raw leafy vegetables
$\frac{1}{2}$ cup cooked or chopped vegetables
$\frac{3}{4}$ cup vegetable juice

Milk, Yogurt, Cheese

1 cup milk or yogurt
$1\frac{1}{2}$ ounce of cheese
2 ounces process cheese

Meat, Poultry, Fish, Dry Beans, Eggs, and Nuts

2–3 ounces of cooked lean meat, poultry, or fish = 1 serving from this food group
$\frac{1}{2}$ cup of cooked dry beans = 1 ounce lean meat
1 egg = 1 ounce lean meat
2 tablespoons peanut butter = 1 ounce lean meat

Food products can belong to one group or can be a combination of two or more groups and provide nutrients from several of the groups on the Pyramid. For example, pizza provides nutrients from the bread and cereal group, the milk and cheese group, and, depending on the topping, from the vegetable or meat group.

Although diet will often be as important to the health of your client as his medication or exercise regime, the client and his family may not understand this. Discuss with your supervisor ways to teach the family the importance of food and the proper diet while incorporating family and cultural preferences. If you do not understand some cultural food practices, you may discuss them with the client or a family member in a respectful and nonjudgmental manner.

THE DIETARY GUIDELINES*

The Dietary Guidelines for Americans can serve as a useful outline for choosing a healthy, balanced diet for good health. These guidelines are recommended for healthy children over the age of 2 years and adults at any age. They can be modified and used by all persons, including those on **prescribed diets** or those who just want to improve overall health. It is important to discuss any change in diet, physical activity, or taking of supplements with your supervisor before the client initiates the change.

There are three basic messages, also known as the ABCs.

- **A**im for fitness
- **B**uild a healthy base
- **C**hoose sensibly

Within these three messages, there are 10 guidelines to follow:

Aim for Fitness

1. Aim for a healthy weight.
   Many Americans start to gain weight in adulthood. Overweight increases your risk for high blood pressure, heart disease, stroke, diabetes, certain types of cancer, arthritis, breathing problems, and other illnesses. Losing just 10 percent of excess weight can have a significant improvement on health. For example, if a person weighs 190 pounds and is overweight, and loses 19 pounds, this can improve overall health.
2. Be physically active each day.
   Physical activity promotes fitness, which improves health. The general recommendation is for at least 30 minutes of physical activity daily. There are many health benefits of physical activity, including managing weight and lowering risk factors for some diseases.

---

*Adapted from the U.S. Department of Agriculture, U.S. Department of Health and Human Services, *Nutrition and Your Health: Dietary Guidelines for Americans* (5th ed.), 2000.

Build a Healthy Base

3. Let the Pyramid guide your food choices.
4. Choose a variety of grains daily, especially whole grains.
5. Choose a variety of fruits and vegetables daily.
6. Keep food safe to eat.

Eating a variety of food is important to obtain nutrients needed for good health. The body needs vitamins, minerals, protein, fat, and carbohydrate. Different nutrients are found in different foods. No single food can supply all nutrients in the amounts you need.

Choose Sensibly

7. Choose a diet that is low in saturated fat and cholesterol and moderate in total fat.
   This guideline emphasizes the continued importance of choosing a diet with less total fat, saturated fat, and cholesterol. It does not suggest eliminating all fat in one's diet.
8. Choose beverages and foods that limit the intake of sugars.
   Examples of sugars are milk, fruits, vegetables, breads, cereals, and grains. Many people like the taste of sugar and add it to foods. The body cannot tell the difference between naturally occurring sugars and sugars that have been added. It is recommended to limit the amount of simple sugars added to foods, not what is naturally occurring in food. These foods items that should be limited include candy, table sugar, soda, and cakes.
9. Choose and prepare foods with less salt.
   Sodium and **sodium chloride,** commonly known as salt, occur naturally in foods, usually in small amounts, and are necessary in small amounts for the body to function properly. Salt and other sodium ingredients are often added to products during food processing. Some people add salt from a shaker or use products high in sodium such as soy sauce. Salt is thought to enhance the flavors of foods. As the amount of salt is lessened, so does the preference for the taste of salt. Excess sodium acts like a sponge holding on to extra fluids in the body. This makes the heart work harder to pump blood throughout the body. Healthy dietary intakes of sodium can range from 2 grams to 5 grams per day.
10. If you drink alcoholic beverages, do so in moderation.
    Alcoholic beverages simply supply calories but no nutrients. **Alcohol** consumed in excess can have harmful effects on judgment and body organs. Alcohol also may interfere with activities that require attention or skill. Continued use of alcohol can lead to dependency on it. Alcohol also interferes with many medica-

tions. A glass of wine with dinner is not prohibited, but all other factors must be considered such as dietary restrictions and use of medications. Pregnant and nursing women should avoid all alcohol during this period.

It is important to understand the message, but following the guidelines will help you stay healthy and fit. Remember the ABCs when planning and selecting food choices.

- **A**im for fitness
- **B**uild a healthy base
- **C**hoose sensibly

VEGETARIANS

Vegetarians eat no animal meat or by-products. Being a vegetarian means different things to different people, but, most commonly, they all eat plant-based diets. Vegetarian diets are often classified by what foods they include. A **vegan** diet is the strictest and only includes plant foods. A **lacto-vegetarian** diet includes dairy products and plant foods. An **Ovo-vegetarian** diet includes eggs and plant foods. A **lacto-ovo-vegetarian** diet includes dairy products, eggs, and plant foods. A **semi-vegetarian** diet excludes red meat, but may include fish or poultry, dairy, eggs, and plant foods. People choose to be vegetarians for different reasons. Some reasons may be cultural beliefs and practices, religious or philosophical beliefs, economic or ecological concerns, or purely interest in health. Whatever the reason, a balanced diet can be maintained and the Food Pyramid used as a guide.

YOUR ROLE AS A HOMEMAKER/HOME HEALTH AIDE

You may notice that one part of the Pyramid is not included in a client's diet. Discuss this with your supervisor so that a supplement or change can be recommended. People who have strong bonds with their ethnic background may choose foods that are not familiar to the homemaker/home health aide. Frequently, clients will not keep to a prescribed diet but eat foods that are more familiar to them. Encourage clients to stay on their **therapeutic diet,** and notify the supervisor if problems are noted. Most of the time, your client's therapeutic diet can be adapted to his or her ethnic preferences. If you are unfamiliar with the dietary habits of your client, discuss this with your supervisor. Then you will learn, and you will be able to help your client within his or her ethnic tradition.

POINTS TO REMEMBER

- Using the Food Pyramid as the basis for meal planning will provide the most comprehensive way to incorporate all nutrients into a diet.
- Variety from the food groups will provide all the nutrients necessary.
- Moderation in all food should be the focus of meal planning. Modification should be based on client need and preference.
- Follow the Dietary Guidelines.
- Respect for cultural food practices should and can be accommodated while still maintaining a nutritious and balanced diet.
- Observe what foods are preferred, eaten, and tolerated well by your client.
- Observe and report food intolerances or avoidances to your supervisor so that the necessary nutrient can be obtained in other forms.

CHAPTER 2

Food Supplements, Herbal Supplements, Vitamins

Introduction

In this chapter, you will become familiar with some of the reasons people take food supplements, herbal supplements, and vitamins. You will explore your role in supporting your clients as they take them as part of their total nutritional program. You will gain familiarity with new words associated with plant chemicals, which are thought to help in the fight against diseases.

Dietary supplements are substances that are thought to improve the action of the food we eat. Dietary supplements of any kind are taken for various reasons:

- Many people believe, even though they are healthy, they must consume dietary supplements because the food that they eat does not contain all the nutrients and micronutrients they need for a healthy body.
- Some people do not consume a well-balanced diet due to disease, preference, habit, or cultural practice and feel the supplements will eliminate the nutritional deficiencies they may have.

- A person requires additional calories and/or nutrients he or she cannot get through food.
- A person requires very detailed and precise monitoring of his or her nutritional intake.
- A person cannot digest regular food.

Dietary supplements include prepared liquids or powders, puddings, minerals, dietary fibers, amino acids, and plant or animal extracts and herbal preparations. They may be taken as capsules, powders, liquids, teas, or pills. They may be taken hot or cold. Most supplements can be purchased without prescription and therefore many health care professionals are not aware that their clients are taking them. It is important that everyone involved in the client's care be aware of all substances the client takes. Encourage your client to share this information with his health care professionals.

Supplements are not a substitute for eating well and maintaining a healthy lifestyle. Eating a variety of food from the Food Pyramid should provide all the nutrients essential for good health making most food supplement unnecessary. If supplements are necessary, they should be prescribed by a reputable health care professional who is knowledgeable about the products being recommended and the client's health history, lifestyle, and medications—both prescription and nonprescription.

Supplements may be prescribed for an extended period of time if the health status of the client is not expected to improve or the condition is deemed **chronic.** Sometimes, supplements may be necessary for a short period of time due to an **acute** health condition that is expected to resolve or improve. Supplements should be taken as prescribed and their intake and effect closely monitored to prevent toxic and negative side effects.

SUPPORTING A CLIENT TAKING SUPPLEMENTS

Support your client and the family as he or she takes the supplements that have been prescribed. Help clients incorporate them into their daily routine. Be sure to note all supplements taken by your client, whether they are prescribed or not and whether they are considered prescription or over-the-counter preparations. If you have reason to believe that a supplement or practice is not safe, report it to your supervisor immediately. You should note the effect of the supplement and objectively report any side effects. Sometimes, a supplement may not interact well with prescription medications. Therefore, it is very important to share with your supervisor all the supplements taken by your client, their effect, and your observations so that it can be determined that there is no adverse interaction and indeed that there is some benefit.

Supplements and herbs usually need no refrigeration until they have been opened. Some people enjoy the supplements better if chilled. Ask your client his or her preference. Some supplements should be mixed with liquid before being taken. It is important to use the correct amount of fluid and the recommended fluid. Do not mix supplements unless you have been instructed to do so by your supervisor.

HERBAL PREPARATIONS AND ANTIOXIDANTS

Herbs have been used as digestive aids, as treatments for diseases, and as preventative substances for thousands of years. They are used differently in different cultures and by different practitioners. Often, herbal preparations are seen as fads and gain popularity and then fade from practice. However, as more and more is learned about the chemical makeup of food and herbs, we may see the increased use and regulation of these preparations.

The preparation of herbs and some dietary supplements is not regulated at this time, however, and the client must rely on the skill and the knowledge of the health care professional. It is important that the health care professional be familiar with the interaction of the herbs with the prescribed medication. Lack of knowledge about these interactions may results in clients taking substances they know very little about with unknown and unexpected effects. Therefore, your objective observations are very important to the total health of your client. Share your observations with your supervisor and the client.

Phytochemicals are substances found in plants that have no nutritional value but are thought to fight against cancer. Phytochemicals can be found in vegetables, fruits, grains, nuts, and seeds. Vitamins C, E, and beta-carotene are examples of phytochemicals known as **antioxidants.** These protect us against harmful cell damage from **oxidation** and are found in fruits and vegetables and thought to protect body tissue against oxygen-induced damage to tissues (Table 2.1).

Different phytochemicals may offer front-line defense against cancer and can be found in broccoli, cabbage, beans, legumes, strawberries, tomato, oranges, tofu, soy milk, and other foods made from soybeans.

Table 2.1 Antioxidant Food Sources	
Beta-carotene and vitamin A	Green leafy vegetables, broccoli, collard greens, kale, spinach, red, orange, and yellow fruit and vegetables; apricots; blueberries; cantaloupe; carrots; mango; papaya; peaches; pumpkin; sweet potatoes; tomatoes; watermelon; winter squash
Vitamin C	Broccoli, cantaloupe, citrus fruits (orange, grapefruit, lemon), kiwi, potatoes, red peppers, strawberries, tomatoes
Vitamin E	Almond, margarine, nuts, seeds, vegetable oil, wheat germ, sunflower seeds

VITAMINS AND MINERALS

Vitamins and minerals are both needed in the body in small amounts. There are 13 known vitamins. They are divided into two classes: water soluble and fat soluble. The water-soluble vitamins include the B vitamins—thiamine (B_1), riboflavin (B_2), niacin (B_3), pyridoxine (B_6), cobalamine (B_{12})—biotin, pantothenic acid, folic acid, and vitamin C. The body absorbs what is needed, and the excess is excreted in the urine. The fat-soluble vitamins are A, D, E, and K. They are stored in body fat. Excess intake will be accumulated in the body. High levels of these vitamins may cause a toxic effect.

Minerals are also important to consume in the diet. Like vitamins, minerals are needed in small amounts. They are found in all foods with the exception of highly refined foods. Some of the more common minerals include calcium, iron, magnesium, potassium, and phosphorus (Table 2.2).

Table 2.2 Vitamins and Minerals

Vitamin/Mineral	Important Functions	Food Sources
Thiamine (vitamin B_1)	Promotes normal appetite and digestion; helps keep healthy nervous system	Meat, fish, poultry; pork supplies about three times as much as other meats. Eggs, dried peas, and beans; peanuts; enriched or whole-grain breads and cereals; potatoes; broccoli; collards; melons
Vitamin A	Helps keep skin clear and smooth; helps resistance to infection; helps prevent night blindness; promotes growth	Carrots, sweet potatoes, yellow vegetables, egg yolks
Niacin (vitamin B_3)	Helps nervous system stay healthy; keeps skin, mouth, tongue, and digestive tract in healthy condition; helps cells in the body use oxygen to produce energy	Peanut butter, meat, fish, poultry, enriched or whole-grain breads and cereals, mushrooms

Table 2.2 *(continued)*

Vitamin/Mineral	Important Functions	Food Sources
Riboflavin (vitamin B_2)	Helps prevent scaly, greasy skin around mouth and nose; helps cells use oxygen to release energy from foods	Milk, ice cream, cheese; meat, especially liver, fish, poultry; eggs; vegetable greens; soybeans; whole-grain or enriched cereal products
Pyridoxine (vitamin B_6)	Used to help nerve tissues function normally; plays an important role in red cell regeneration; used in metabolism of amino acids, fats, and carbohydrate	Dairy products, pork, soybeans, beef liver, legumes, bananas, whole-grain cereals, sweet potatoes, white potatoes
Cobalamine (vitamin B_{12})	Needed to prevent development of pernicious anemia	Eggs, fish, liver, meats, milk
Folacin or folic acid	Needed for regulation of red blood cells	Eggs, beef, vegetable greens, whole-grain or enriched cereals
Pantothenic acid	Helps with transmission of nerve impulses; helps with utilization of energy	Eggs, meats, milk, organ meats, peanuts, whole-grain or enriched products
Vitamin C	Helps in healing wounds and broken bones; strengthens walls of the blood vessels; helps teeth and bone formation	Citrus fruits, tomatoes, strawberries, melons, potatoes, green vegetables
Vitamin D	Helps the body use calcium and phosphorus to build strong bones and teeth	Egg yolk, vitamin D–fortified milk, fish liver oil; plenty of sunshine, not food
Vitamin E	Maintains functioning of skeletal muscle, brain, and blood cells; has a role in reproduction, protects vitamin A and carotene from destruction by oxidation	Liver, eggs, milk, green leafy vegetables, vegetable oils, nuts and legumes

continues

Table 2.2 *(continued)*

Vitamin/Mineral	Important Functions	Food Sources
Vitamin K	Maintains normal clotting functions of the blood	Green leafy vegetables, cauliflower, vegetable oil, cabbage, tomatoes
Calcium	Helps build strong bones and teeth; helps the blood to clot; regulates heartbeat; helps muscles and nerves to work; helps regulate the use of other minerals in the body	Milk, cheeses, turnips, mustard greens, collards, kale, broccoli
Iron	Combines with protein to help carry oxygen to the cells; helps cells use oxygen	Meats, dried beans, green leafy vegetables, prunes, raisins, enriched or whole-grain breads and cereals
Magnesium	Helps with bone growth and lipid metabolism	Most dairy products excluding butter, flour and flour products, dry beans and peas, soybeans, nuts, vegetable greens
Potassium	Helps maintain fluid balance; helps with transmission of impulses	Bananas, potatoes, bran, apricots, avocado, dried fruits, prunes, prune juice, wheat germ, milk, coffee
Phosphorus	Helps build bones and teeth; helps regulate many internal activities in the body	Liver, fish, poultry, eggs, milk, cheeses, whole-grain cereals, nuts and legumes

YOUR ROLE AS A HOMEMAKER/HOME HEALTH AIDE

The total nutrition of your clients will include everything they eat and drink, including prescribed and nonprescribed supplements and herbs. By becoming familiar with all the products, prescribed diet, and your client's personal likes and dislikes, you will be able to work with your supervisor and the client and his or her family to create a dietary plan that is pleasing to your client. It is important that your supervisor be aware of any supplements, herbs, or vitamins taken by your client. You may have to explain to your clients that the reason you are sharing this information with your supervisor is not to tell on them, but rather to ensure their safety and health. Continue to encourage your clients to gain information from all sources but to discuss this information with their health care professional before they change their dietary regime.

POINTS TO REMEMBER

- Food supplement, herbal preparations, and vitamins should be prescribed by a physician.
- Some supplements do not interact well with prescription medicines. Observation of the effect of all supplements on the client is an important role of the homemaker/home health aide.
- Food supplements are not substitutes for a balanced intake of food but are designed to enhance regular food.
- Supplements should be incorporated into the regular diet.

CHAPTER 3
Feeding a Client

Introduction

In this chapter, you will become familiar with the many factors you must consider when preparing to feed and feeding a client. You will become familiar with the factors associated with feeding adults and children, whether they are your client or members of the family. Finally, you will become familiar with activities that contribute to a pleasant, safe, and meaningful experience for a client or family member who must be fed.

At about the age of 2 or 3 years, children are taught to feed themselves. Their skill with forks and knives continues to improve with age. Although an adult may have to cut meat or help the child, children are soon feeding themselves. In American culture, it is an expectation that people will feed themselves. Usually, eating is a pleasurable activity with one or more people. Each person adopts some activities that are associated with eating. Some people always sit in the same seat at the table. Some people always read during a meal, while others like to listen to music. These activities contribute to the total eating experience. It is important that these activities be honored even if the client cannot perform all of them. Make mealtime fun and an enjoyable experience for the client.

When the ability to feed oneself is compromised or diminished, someone else must provide that service. Sometimes, the feeding of a client is shared among family members. Sometimes, it becomes the responsibility of one person. Although feeding oneself is done without much thought, feeding others requires a great deal of consideration and planning. Remember that your clients, whether they are adults or children, may feel embarrassed or uncomfortable that they cannot feed themselves.

Assisting a Client with Feeding

Some clients cannot feed themselves because:

- They are too weak.
- They cannot safely move the food from the plate or glass to their mouth.
- They cannot swallow safely and therefore cannot eat alone.
- They have temporary or permanent physical limitations.
- They have a cognitive or mental limitation and cannot remember to eat or complete a meal.

Planning to Feed a Client

Planning meals is very important. For some clients, planning regular meals is necessary from a health perspective; for some people, it is due to personal habits. Some people like to eat several small meals a day. Some people like to snack.

Everyone has some habits associated with eating that are important to them. Some habits are cultural, some are related to health, and some just contribute to the comfort level of the person. It is important to find out as much as possible about your clients' habits concerning eating. You will then be able to plan to meet their needs and make eating a pleasant, desirable experience. Listed below are some common questions to help you get acquainted with clients whether they are adults or children.

- Where does the client usually eat? Can the client continue to eat there or must the place be changed? Why?
- Does the client usually eat alone?
- Are all meals eaten the same way? In the same place?
- Does the client usually watch television, read, or listen to the radio when eating?
- Does the client wash his or her hands and face before eating?
- Does the client wear a special garment while eating?
- Does the client like hot liquids? Hot food? Cold liquids? Cold food?
- Does the client enjoy eating the meal in a particular order?
- Are there any prescribed therapeutic dietary restrictions?
- Are there any self- or family imposed dietary restrictions?
- Are there any religious dietary restrictions? Does the client wish to follow them?
- Is the client allergic to any foods?

- Are there any foods the client states bothers him or her if eaten?
- Are there any food–drug interactions that must be considered?
- What is the extent of the client's limitations? Can he or she take part in any of the activities associated with feeding and mealtime?
- Can the client swallow all food? Liquids? Solids?
- Is the client's condition expected to change? Improve? Deteriorate?
- Can the client communicate? At what level?
- Ask the client if there is anything else he or she would like you to know regarding feeding or mealtimes.

Getting the information you need *before* you start to feed a client may take some creativity. You may have to ask your supervisor, family members, or the client and rely on your observational skills. Be sure to clarify and validate your findings with the family and the client. Do not assume anything. Review your final plan with the client if at all possible before you start a meal. Sharing your plans prepares the client and indicates your concern and consideration for his or her needs and preferences. Remember that the client's feelings regarding feeding can change from day to day. Be sure to have this conversation as often as necessary.

Basic Considerations

- Do not rush the feeding.
- Provide a safe, pleasant environment acceptable to the client.
- Offer the client the use of the bathroom or bedpan before the meal starts.
- Be sure the client's hands are clean.
- If appropriate, offer the client mouth care before and after the meal.
- Speak to the client in **age-appropriate** language.
- Serve foods the client enjoys eating.
- Do not argue or force a client to eat.
- Do not use food as a reward or a punishment.
- Use feeding time as a special social time.
- Encourage the client to be part of meal planning.

Physical Limitations

Providing assistance and **assistive devices** to clients can often improve their ability to feed themselves. Often, clients with physical limitations

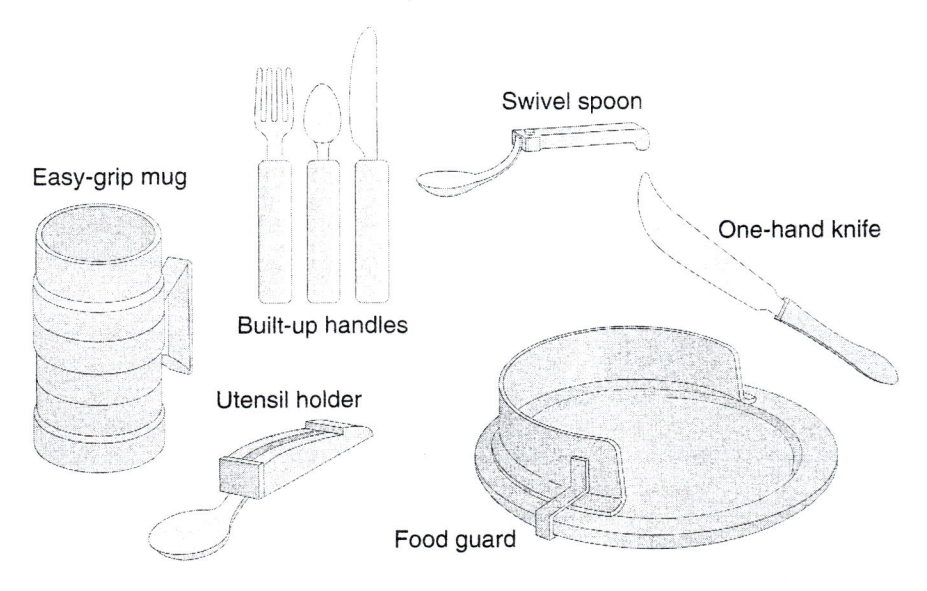

FIGURE 3.1 Utensils designed to assist clients in eating.

can make use of specially designed utensils, which will increase their independence. For instance, plates with rims and forks with large handles may help the client (Figure 3.1). Discuss with the client, the family, and your supervisor the use of some these aids. Everyone accepts these aids differently, so planning their introduction into the home is something that should be carefully considered. Remember, most people like to feed themselves.

SAFETY FACTORS

Be sure a client is able to swallow both liquids and solid foods before you put food in his or her mouth or on the plate. Some clients will be able to swallow one food but not another. Some clients say they can swallow but are unable to completely empty their mouths. Your observation is very important. If a client has weakness on one side of his or her mouth, place the food in the **unaffected side.** Pay special attention to the temperature of the food. If food is hot, tell the client and then offer small amounts. If the food is cold, do the same. Never feed clients while they are lying down.

If the client is blind, name each mouthful before you offer it him or her. Describe the items on the plate and their placement. Some clients may wish to touch the food. Assist with this as necessary (Figure 3.2).

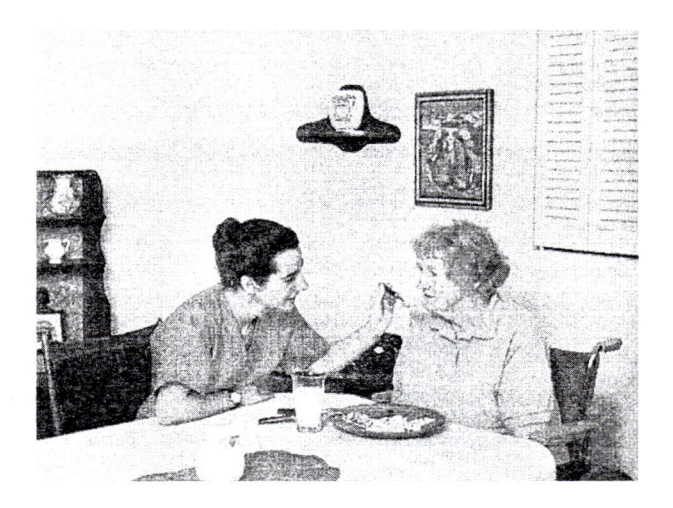

FIGURE 3.2 Feed a client in a quiet atmosphere. Both you and the client should be comfortable.

While feeding clients, continually observe them. Be sure that all food has been swallowed. If the client is tired, wait until he or she is ready to eat again. Do not ask questions of clients while they have food in their mouth (Figure 3.3). Do not leave clients alone while they are chewing or swallowing. Be sure to review with your supervisor your response if a client appears to be choking. Be sure you know how to respond if you are feeding an adult or a child.

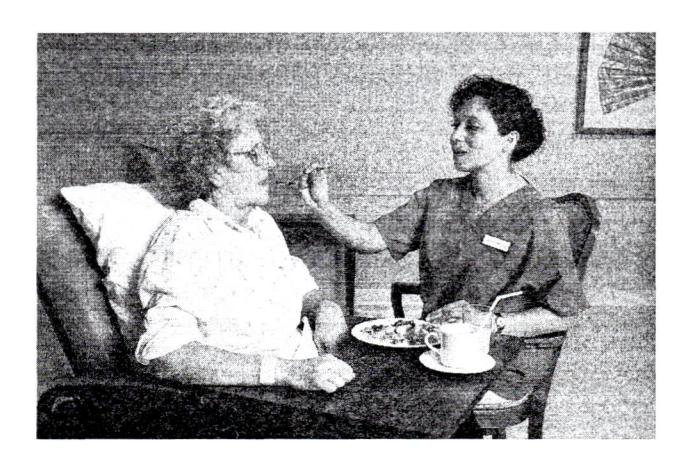

FIGURE 3.3 Assist a client in bed to eat in an upright position and in a safe relaxed manner.

Feeding Children **25**

FEEDING CHILDREN

Children are fed differently at different ages. Sometimes when a child is ill or there is illness in the home, a child will revert to behavior of a younger child. Do not become alarmed unless this behavior continues. Then report it to your supervisor. It is important that you find out how the child is usually fed. If it is safe and the child seems to respond well, you should maintain the same routine the child is used to and the household can support. If you see changes that would improve the nutritional content of the meals, the routine associated with eating, or the preparation of the food, discuss this with your supervisor and work with the family to institute the changes. Do not make sweeping changes without discussing them with the mother of the child or the main caregiver.

Nutritional habits are shaped early in a child's life. Keep the following facts in mind as you review the child's eating habits:

- Appetites change and so does food intake. Some days, children will eat more than on other days. Some days, children will eat by themselves, and other days they may want to be fed. Some days, they will eat a great deal, and other days they will not. Do not become alarmed unless you see changes such as weight, abilities, sleep changes, or mood changes. Report these to your supervisor immediately.
- Children eat small amounts of food frequently. Children under the age of 6 usually have at least two to three snacks a day. This food, eaten between regular meals, is a necessary source of nutrition and calories for the child. The snacks should be nutritionally valuable, such as fruit, cheese, raw vegetables, yogurt, and whole-grain crackers.
- All activities in the home influence food intake, especially family dynamics, available food, social environment, illness, and the attitudes of the family members toward children.
- Activities associated with food and eating are important factors in developing attitudes toward food.
- What are the expectations of the child during feeding? How much the child should eat, use of utensils, length of time at the table, and the child's role at the table all influence the child's attitudes toward food, eating, and nutritional content.

Every child grows and develops at a different pace. It is important to remember that each child is unique. It is also important to remember that children may change their usual habits when they have a new caretaker, when they are ill, or when there is someone in the household who is ill and normal routines are changed. Your role is to make mealtime a pleasant experience. Offer food in a relaxed and giving manner. Never use food in the disciplinary process. If you become aware that other family members withhold food as a part of discipline, report this to your supervisor immediately.

Table 3.1 should be used as a *guide* when determining how much to feed a child.

A general guide for preparing food for children is to offer about one tablespoon of a food for every year of age. Also take into consideration the child's likes and dislikes and his or her general appetite. Another way to think of the amount of food is:

- A child between the ages of 2 and 3 usually can start with one fourth the amount of an adult portion.
- A preschooler 4 to 5 years old: one half the amount of an adult portion.
- A young school-age child: three fourths of an adult portion.

Table 3.1 Suggested Servings and Portion Sizes for Children

Food Group	Servings per Day[a]	Food Item	Toddler	Pre-schooler	6–8 Year Old
Grains—bread, cereal, rice, pasta (base of pyramid)	6	Bread Pasta or rice Cereal—cold or hot	¼–½ slice ¼ cup ¼ cup	½ slice ⅓ cup ⅓ cup	1 slice ½ cup ½ cup
Vegetables	3	Vegetables—cooked or raw	2 Tbsp	¼ cup	½ cup
Fruits	2	Fruits—fresh Fruit—canned Fruit juice	2 Tbsp ¼ cup ¼ cup	¼ cup ½ cup ½ cup	1 medium ½ cup ½ cup
Dairy—milk, yogurt, and cheeses	3–4	Milk or yogurt Cheese	½ cup 1 ounce	¾ cup 1½ ounces	1 cup 1½–2 ounces
Meat, poultry, fish, beans, eggs	2–3	Meat, poultry, fish Cooked beans Eggs Peanut butter	1 ounce 2 Tbsp ½ 1 Tbsp	1½ ounce ¼ cup 1 2 Tbsp	2–3 ounces ½ cup 1 2 Tbsp

[a] *Servings per day is intended as a guideline. Some may need more servings based on caloric needs.*

Table 3.2

Age	Skill	Tips
0–6 months	Totally dependent on adults for food; solid food may be introduced but not before 4 months of age. Schedule changes frequently due to changes in his sleep pattern; cannot control his head well; sleeps about 14–16 hours a day.	Be sure the baby is in a comfortable, safe position; do not prop his bottle; always hold the baby when feeding him a bottle; be alert to allergic reactions as new foods are introduced; place the small baby spoon inside his lips and let him suck the food off it; do not put the food too far back in the baby's mouth as this will cause him to gag. After feeding 2–4 ounces, burp baby.
6–12 months	Solid food introduced; may start to handle a cup; puts everything in his mouth; may start to feed himself; displays likes and dislikes; sleeps about 10 hours at night and has two naps a day of about 1–2 hours.	Offer foods in relaxed manner. Observe child while eating. Never leave child unattended while eating. Encourage finger feeding. (See Table 3.3 for foods to avoid.)
1–2 years	Primarily uses fingers to eat; may pick up only certain foods; puts everything in his mouth; has very short attention span; may still have two naps a day but shorter.	Sit child at table for meals and snack; use unbreakable dishes and cups; use special spoon with wide bowl for children; child will learn to use spoon before he uses a fork; cut food into small pieces. (See Table 3.3 for foods to avoid.)
2–3 years	Uses a cup; learns to use a straw; wants to do everything himself; uses a spoon well; will imitate those around them when eating; usually naps only in the afternoon.	Eats frequently; snacks are necessary; encourage use of cup for drinking; can introduce new foods accompanied by familiar ones; responds well to colorful foods. Start discussing nutritional value of food: Insist child eats sitting down. (See Table 3.3 for foods to avoid.)
4–5 years	Likes to choose his food; likes to eat with others, especially adults; understands the concept of waiting for food; responds well to consistent expectations from all adults; does not nap on a regular basis.	Allow children to take part in choosing and preparing food; remind them of expectations at mealtime; can imitate good table manners; introduce new foods slowly and with realistic expectations.

Physical Abilities of Children

The physical abilities of a child influence how and what a child is fed. At different ages, there are different general expectations for what and how children eat. Table 3.2 is a guide. If you have concerns about a child in your care, discuss these concerns with your supervisor, reporting objective observations in a timely manner.

Children should not run or play with food in their mouth. Children have problems grinding and chewing some foods because they may not have all their teeth. Children often choke on foods that are tough, hard to chew, round, small, long, or sticky. These foods should be avoided unless extreme caution is used (Table 3.3).

Teething and rub-on medications can cause problems with chewing and swallowing. It can cause the muscles in the throat to become **numb**. If these products are used, close observation is necessary during the feeding period.

Cleaning Up

When a client is finished eating, you can assist the client with returning to his or her regular activities. As you clean up the eating area, notice and document the foods that were eaten and not eaten, and indicate the amounts. Make a note of anything else that happened during the meal, such as the client's ability to swallow, or discussions about the client's family or ability to feed him- or herself. Discuss these observations with your supervisor.

Table 3.3 Foods to Avoid for Children

Corn
Nuts
Popcorn
Hard sucking candy
Raw vegetables
Frankfurters, unless they are skinless and cut into small pieces
Grapes
Peas
Peanut butter, unless it is in a sandwich with jelly
Spaghetti, unless it is cut into small pieces

Your Role as a Homemaker/Home Health Aide

It is often difficult to decide whether you will actually feed clients or you will assist them as they eat. Sometimes it is easier to ask clients what they prefer. Involve them in the decision if at all possible. You may find that they like to eat some foods themselves but need assistance with others. You may find that their needs change with each meal. Your role is to determine the client's needs and meet them in an age-appropriate manner. As you do this, you will ensure a safe and dignified environment for the client. Share your observations with the family so they too can assist the client when you are not in the home.

POINTS TO REMEMBER

- Gather as much information about clients, their habits and preferences, and their abilities before you plan mealtime. Be sure to discuss your plans with clients before you finalize them.
- Feeding a client is a very personal activity associated with many personal practices, which must be honored.
- Safety is an important part of feeding time. Be observant to client abilities and react to them in a timely manner. Discuss your observations with your supervisor.
- Make mealtime an enjoyable experience.
- Children's appetites vary, so offer them a variety of food in small amounts appropriate for their age.

CHAPTER 4
Cultural Aspects of Food

Introduction

In this chapter, you will learn about the many different things that influence the food we eat and the food we do not eat. As each **culture** *developed, food preferences and beliefs became part of their everyday life. Respect for these beliefs and practices is essential as you work with your clients.*

Human beings are able to eat both animal and vegetable matter. This ability evolved slowly over millions of years. Through trial and error, people discovered that even certain vegetable matter like grass and leaves were not good to eat and very hard to digest. But they also discovered that other vegetables like carrots, potatoes, and nuts were easy to eat, easy to store, and had a taste that was pleasant.

After a forest fire, when the fire killed animals such as deer and bear, it is thought that someone discovered that the flesh tasted good cooked. This accident of discovery probably led to the practice of roasting meat and even some vegetables. By cooking the meat, it was tastier, easier to store, and easier to transport as the groups of people moved about. Thus, people began to develop preferences for certain foods and preparation of these foods.

INFLUENCES ON FOOD CHOICES

Many things influence and effect food habits of groups of people and of individuals. Throughout history the changes were very slow. Now, however, the changes are much faster.

- Travel has been and continues to be a prime influence on food choices. Travel due to war, weather changes, or pleasure has taken people to many places. As people went from one country or area of the world to another, they adapted food to their culture. As people travel today, they bring back food, recipes, and spices to their own table.

- Religious practices influence what is eaten and how it is eaten. Some cultures do not eat beef. In some Jewish households, a **kosher** kitchen may be kept. This means that utensils and equipment used for meat products must be kept separately from those used for dairy products. Meat and dairy may not be eaten at the same meal. Pork and shellfish products are never eaten. The degree to which a client keeps a kosher home varies and should be discussed with the family. Some ethnic groups may not eat pork or shellfish but do not keep a kosher home. Some people require that their meat be slaughtered according to religious practices. Some people are vegetarians as prescribed by their religious beliefs. The impact these beliefs and practices have on the prescribed diet should be discussed with your supervisor.
- Economic status affects tastes in food. If a food is so expensive that only the very wealthy can afford it, that food substance becomes known as a "rich man's food," and recipes of the common people will not contain it. If food is inexpensive or easy to grow, it gains in popularity. Your clients will bring these beliefs with them, and they will influence their choice of foods and the way they are prepared.
- Storage of food has always been a challenge. Food that is easily stored, such as grains, roots, and dried meat, became staples of cultures that did not have the ability to continually obtain more food. These people had to get it when they could and keep it fresh until they needed it. Thus, certain foods were eaten in summer, others in winter, and some year round, depending on storage and availability. Fruit, which was difficult to grow and perishable, was often eaten only by the rich. However, in warmer climates, this may not have been true.
- Processing of food such as grains, cheese, and some meat was very labor intensive and often not available to everyone. Therefore, only the very rich could afford to have white flour; cheese, which took months or even years to make; or meat, which had to be slaughtered and kept fresh.
- Natural availability heavily influenced food habits. People living near lakes, streams, and oceans naturally used fish as a source of protein, while people living inland and away from water developed eating habits that did not include fish.
- Superstition may dictate some practices that have been handed down from one generation to another. These may make people feel safe or connected to their past.

- Traditionally, certain foods may be prepared by men or women. Although no one will be able to tell you exactly why, they will say, "It has always been that way."

How We Eat

All cultures do not eat the same way. The practices grew up over a very long period of time and may not have changed. They originally may have been established to meet a need that no longer exists, but the practice continues. How food is eaten is as important as what is eaten. Eating and sharing of food has always been a group activity and had special social meaning to the participants and other members of the group. It is important that this meaning be maintained unless the family or client wishes it changed (Figure 4.1).

- Do people eat at a table with chairs?
- Who eats and who serves the food?
- Do the women and men eat together?
- When and where do the children eat?
- Do people use utensils?
- Does someone say a blessing before the eating begins?
- Is there a general area where people eat?
- Is the eating area prepared in a special way before eating?
- Is there a special order in which food is served?
- Are there special seats for certain people?

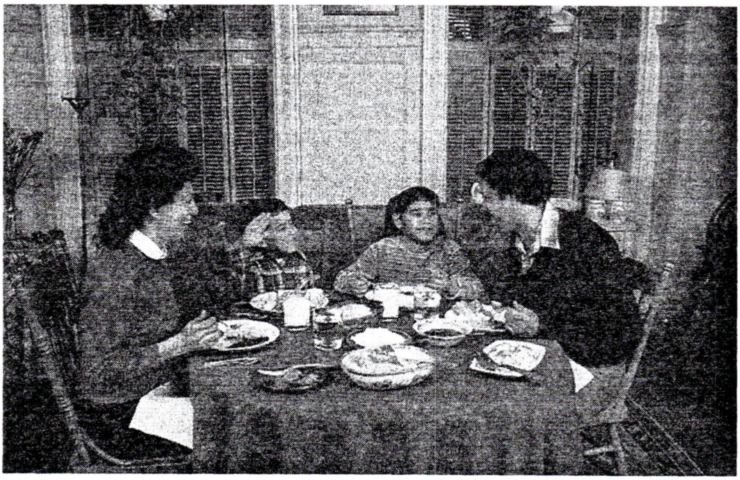

FIGURE 4.1 Eating together provides family members with time to share experiences.

Changing What We Eat

Changing habits, even if we want to, is very difficult. Everyone makes changes for different reasons. Some of the more common reasons that motivate change are:

- New knowledge
- Fear of dying or becoming ill again
- Positive reinforcement from family or important people
- Financial incentives
- Religious practices
- Changing tastes
- Food intolerances
- Changes in role within the family

Changing Is Difficult

There are several reasons people do not change their behaviors. Identifying the reason(s) is often difficult. But it is helpful to try and identify the reasons as they shed light on our behaviors:

- Religious reasons
- Role in the family unit changes
- The change costs too much
- Disbelief that the change is important
- Lack of family support
- Lack of understanding
- Lack of importance

Your Role as a Homemaker/Home Health Aide

As you enter a house, it very important to remember that the practices surrounding food preparation and eating have been in place for many years and have many cultural values attached to them. Your role is to find out through observation and tactful questions how these practices affect your client. Often, you will not be familiar with some of the family practices. You may even think they are strange. Be respectful of them, however. Remember, when you are no longer in the house, the client will have to remain with the family. Your primary role is to assist with establishing a nutritional program, which will fit within the family unit and meet the client's needs.

You may be asked to help a client change eating habits. Remember, these habits were established in childhood and continue in other members of the family. This may be very difficult for your client. *Be sensitive.* Your role is to be supportive and reinforce positive behaviors and help explain to the family and client reasons for the changes. If you notice that your client is not following the diet, is important to try and find out the reason. Sometimes, clients will not change their eating habits no matter how you explain the reasons and try to facilitate a change. Report this to your supervisor and respect the client's decision.

Be sure to discuss with your supervisor your observations and your client's adherence to the prescribed diet. If you observe practices that you think are unsafe for the client or put the client in danger, report them to your supervisor immediately.

POINTS TO REMEMBER

- Eating habits and food preferences are part of our culture, family practices, and preferences that have been established over many years and generations.
- Changes in eating habits are possible but take time and understanding.
- Changes in eating habits must have value to clients and be easy to maintain within their family unit.
- Implement one change at a time if possible. This will help the client adjust and accept the change.
- Positive reinforcement from the family and you is imperative if change is to be accomplished and maintained.

CHAPTER 5
Kitchen Staples

Introduction

In this chapter, you will become acquainted with items that are considered **staples** *in a kitchen and your role in maintaining them. By using the checklists, you will identify items that are usual in the home, items that will have to be purchased, and items that are already available for you to use. This will enable you to become familiar with the kitchen and will familiarize you with the items that are culturally unique to this family.*

Whenever a meal is planned, certain items will be identified as being needed. Some of the ingredients will have to be purchased. These items may be those that are perishable, those that are unusual, or those that the cook does not usually keep in the kitchen. There are, however, many items that are considered staples; that is, they are usually in the kitchen and the cook can plan on their being there. Keeping frequently used items, those that are easily stored, and those that are used in small amounts each time, such as spices, shortens the shopping list and makes cooking easier. Several factors determine what is a staple and what is not:

- The amount of room in the kitchen and the rest of the house for storage
- The cooking habits of the client and the family
- Dietary restrictions
- Prescribed diets
- The cultural background of the client and family members
- The financial capabilities of the client and family
- The presence or absence of refrigeration

Different households regard different items as staples. Each household is different. In some households, ketchup, curry, and sesame oil are frequently used, whereas in some homes, you will have to purchase them specifically if they are called for in a recipe.

It is important that you and your client agree on:

- Which items are considered staples and which are not
- The number and size of each item that is usually kept
- Where staples are kept
- The system present in the home for identifying items that must be replenished

*D*ETERMINING THE STAPLES FOR YOUR CLIENT

It is helpful to review the staples in a home by dividing them into the areas where they are stored: the refrigerator (Table 5.1), freezer (Table 5.2), spice rack (Table 5.3), or pantry (Table 5.4). Use Tables 5.1 through

Table 5.1 Refrigerator Staples

Item	Yes/No	# To Purchase	Notes
Butter/margarine			
Cheese: cottage, ricotta, Swiss, Parmesan, American, mozzarella			
Eggs			
Fruit: fresh or canned if opened			
Jelly			
Juices			
Ketchup			
Lemon juice			
Mayonnaise			
Milk			
Mustard			
Salad dressing			
Salad greens			
Vegetables cut up and ready to eat			
Vegetables—fresh			
Yogurt			

Table 5.2 Freezer Staples

Item	Yes/No	# To Purchase	Notes
Assorted cooked items			
Assorted raw meats			
Chopped onions			
Frozen yogurt			
Ground turkey, chicken, or beef			
Ice cream			
Juice			
Rolls/bread			
Sherbet			

Table 5.3 Herbs and Spices

Item	Yes/No	# To Purchase	Notes
Basil			
Bay leaves			
Chili powder			
Cinnamon			
Curry			
Dill			
Garlic powder			
Ginger			
Hot pepper			
Onion powder			
Oregano			
Paprika			
Parsley			
Pepper: ground, whole			
Rosemary			
Sage			
Salt			
Thyme			

Table 5.4 Pantry Staples

Item	Yes/No	# To Purchase	Notes
Bouillon cubes			
Bread crumbs: seasoned, unseasoned			
Canned broth			
Canned fruit			
Canned soups			
Canned tomato sauce, paste			
Canned tomatoes			
Chicken canned in water			
Coffee: instant, ground, decaffeinated, regular			
Crackers			
Dry cereal			
Flour: all purpose, whole wheat			
Milk: dry, nonfat, evaporated, condensed			
Oil: olive, corn, vegetable, cannola, safflower			
Pancake/biscuit mix			
Pasta			
Pearl barley			
Rice cakes			
Rice: long grain, brown, short grain, instant			
Soy sauce, low salt			
Sugar			
Tea: regular, decaffeinated, herb			
Tuna: packed in oil or water, albacore, chunk, light			
Vinegar: white, wine, balsamic			

5.4 as a starting point for discussion with your client. Compare these lists with the staples your client already has and you will create a shopping list and become familiar with the contents of the kitchen and the likes and dislikes of your client all at the same time. When an item is indicated as needed, discuss the size and the number of the items to be purchased. Remember to ask if a **brand name** the client likes is necessary when selecting the item. The food items in each table are arranged alphabetically for your convenience. In the notes section, you can record whether low fat or another variety is necessary. For example, if low-fat yogurt or low-fat cheeses are necessary for your client, it is important to note this. The blanks on the bottom of each table are for you to add whatever the client considers a stable. This could be based on food or cultural preferences.

YOUR ROLE AS A HOMEMAKER/HOME HEALTH AIDE

Most clients will have some staples in their house. You will be a part of determining what additional items to purchase. Keep in mind what the client actually needs. Not everyone needs the same staples in the house. Be sensitive to clients' financial constraints and personal preferences. This will indicate the fact that you care and are individualizing your plan and your shopping list. Guiding clients to make a reasonable decision should be based on their needs, the kind of food they will eat, and the way the food will be prepared.

POINTS TO REMEMBER

➢ Each client will consider different items as staples. Space, finances, culture, tradition, and dietary needs and preferences will determine these items.
➢ Identify those items in the home that are not used and, if the client agrees, dispose of them.
➢ Purchase sizes and numbers of items that are agreeable to the client.
➢ Store recently purchased items behind like items that are already in the home.
➢ Maintain a current list of staples for each home.

CHAPTER 6

Shopping for Food and Reading the Food Label

Introduction

In this chapter, you will become familiar with the way to organize your client's food needs so that you will be able to purchase the most economical food to meet these needs. The whole process—from taking inventory to planning a menu, to writing a shopping list, to reading a food label at the store—will be explored.

As the homemaker/home health aide, you may find it necessary to purchase food for the client. Shopping for food is usually an activity that each person has personalized. Some people shop with a list. Some people shop with a menu. Some people shop once a week and some shop every day. Some people purchase certain items in special stores. It is always important to discuss with the client or the family how they usually shop and try to adhere to their practices as best you can. If you feel you must change something, it is always wise to discuss the changes before you make them.

There are several steps to take, which will ensure that you buy the correct items for the food you plan to cook in the desired amounts in the preferred store.

BEFORE YOU GET TO THE STORE

1. *Plan a menu.* Take into consideration the client's diet, cultural preferences, and ability to swallow, as well as storage space, how many meals you will be preparing, and for how

many meals you are shopping. Take into consideration the recommended servings from the Food Pyramid. Be sure that you discuss this with the client and the family. When planning a meal, remember cost. Most clients are not free to spend an unlimited amount of money on their food, so plan meals that are within their budgets and do not cause waste.

2. *Review the items that are in the pantry, the refrigerator, and the freezer.* This will allow you to identify those items that you need to cook and those items you need to purchase to prepare food or foods on the menu.

3. *Develop a list of what foods will be needed in the home.* You may use your staples list as a guide. Shopping with a list will help avoid unnecessary trips to the store for forgotten ingredients. It will also prevent duplicate buying of foods already on hand and, if grouped by types of food, avoid extra steps in the market This is the time to discuss the sizes of the food and the store the client usually goes to for each item. If you notice an unusual item on the list, it is a good idea to know what the client usually buys when a particular item is unavailable.

4. *It is important to know how you will pay for the groceries.* If the family gives you money, be sure you count it and you both acknowledge how much money you were given. If there is another method of payment, be sure you and the client both are comfortable with it.

At the Store

Shopping in an unfamiliar store is often difficult. It is usually a good idea to take a minute and review the layout of the store. First, shop for nonperishable and pantry food items. These items do not require refrigeration and are not frozen. Then shop for vegetables. Refrigerated items and frozen food foods should be put into your basket right before checkout. Often, the supermarket is not laid out in a manner that makes this order easy. Try to adhere to this order and to minimize the time refrigerated and frozen foods are in the basket.

- Do not choose any meat, poultry, fish, or milk products that feel warm to the touch or packages that are torn or damaged.
- Choose only **pasteurized** dairy products.
- Check eggs to ensure that they are not cracked or dirty.
- Always check the dates on all items. Some are listed as "sell by"; others will say "use by." Select items with the latest dates available.
- When selecting canned products, be sure that cans are not bulging, leaking, or dented on the seam or rim.

Unit Pricing

Unit pricing is a tool available to help the consumer make wise purchases. Unit pricing tells the customer what the cost is by a particular quantity. This can be determined by weight (e.g., a box of cereal might read 72 cents per pound) or by pieces (e.g., a bag of snack bars might read 25 cents per bar). This information is given in addition to the amount you will be charged for the product at the checkout counter. The unit price can be displayed in a variety of ways.

- On a poster that tells all the prices for the food in this section of the store
- By a label on the edge of the shelf where the food is displayed
- On the price sticker that is put on each item

Convenience foods (foods with some of the preparation already done) generally cost more than those made from scratch. If only one or two people are eating the food, however, purchasing the ingredients may result in some of them spoiling before they are completely used. The decision as to whether to purchase ingredients or prepared foods must be made on an individual basis by the client. You can share your opinion, but the client must make the final decision.

Purchasing larger quantities of an item is generally cheaper than buying small quantities. If the item is rarely used or if storage is difficult, however, it may have to be discarded before it is finished and the purchase of the larger quantity may not be the most economical decision. Discuss this with your client before you go to the store so you will not have to make this decision in the store.

Reading a Food Label

(Figure 6.1)

- Daily Value shows how the amount listed compares to that in the **reference diet,** which is usually a 2,000-calorie diet.
- % Daily Value of cholesterol shows how the amount listed in a serving of this food compares to the recommended limit of 300 milligrams, which is the daily value for cholesterol regardless of the calorie level.
- % Daily Value for fiber shows the amount of dietary fiber in a serving of this food compared to the recommended 25 grams for the reference diet of 2,000 calories.
- % Daily Value for vitamin C shows how the amount of vitamin C in a serving of this food compares to the 60-milligram the daily value for vitamin C at all calorie levels.

Not a Low Calorie Food

Nutrition Facts

Serving Size 1 cup (49g)
Servings Per Container about 10

Amount Per Serving	Cereal	Cereal with 1/2 cup Skim Milk
Calories	170	210
Calories from Fat	5	5
	% Daily Value**	
Total Fat 0.5g*	1%	1%
Saturated Fat 0g	0%	0%
Polyunsaturated Fat 0g		
Monounsaturated Fat 0g		
Cholesterol 0mg	0%	0%
Sodium 0mg	0%	3%
Potassium 200mg	6%	11%
Total Carbohydrate 41g	14%	16%
Dietary Fiber 5g	21%	21%
Insoluble Fiber 5g		
Sugars 0g		
Other Carbohydrate 36g		
Protein 5g		
Vitamin A	0%	4%
Vitamin C	0%	2%
Calcium	2%	15%
Iron	8%	8%
Thiamin	8%	10%
Riboflavin	2%	10%

FIGURE 6.1 Learning to read food labels will help you plan meals and budget money.

STRETCHING THE FOOD DOLLAR

Foods in season are almost always a good buy. Menus should be planned with seasonal foods in mind. The cost will be less and the selection greater.

In selecting foods, the best quality is not always necessary. In choosing tomatoes for a salad, the most attractive and usually the most costly would be desirable. However, in selecting tomatoes for tomato sauce, a less expensive tomatoes with a blemish on the skin might be considered a better buy. When selecting foods, you must consider how it will be used and when it will be used in order to make the best decision.

When buying foods high in protein, you can reduce the cost per serving by:

- Using poultry when it is cheaper than meat
- Considering cuts of meat that may cost more per pound but give more servings per person
- Learning to prepare less tender cuts of meat in casseroles or pot roasts
- Serving eggs or egg substitutes
- Substituting dried bean and pea dishes for higher-cost meats
- Using fillers such as bread crumbs or pasta to make a meat dish serve more people

WHEN YOU RETURN HOME

- Put away your groceries away immediately, especially the frozen and refrigerated items. If you are forced to put things in a place other than the one usually used by the family, tell them.
- Review with the client and the family what you bought as well as any substitutions you may have made and the reasons. This is the time to identify those items you did not buy and start a new shopping list.
- Give the family all the change and the receipt so they will have a record of the purchases and the money they spent.
- Document the amount of money spent and the change given the family.

YOUR ROLE AS A HOMEMAKER/HOME HEALTH AIDE

It is sometimes difficult to shop for others, but if you have a detailed list, have discussed with the client exactly what you will buy, and are familiar with the client's diet, you will find it easier. It is wise not to try and save time by doing your personal shopping at the same time. Concentrate on the client's needs. You will make fewer mistakes. You are responsible for giving the client and the family a detailed report of your trip. Note anything you did not buy so that someone else may purchase it. Read the label each time you purchase an item because manufacturers often change ingredients.

POINTS TO REMEMBER

➢ Plan your shopping trip in consultation with the client so that you may purchase the correct items as well as the quantities and sizes of items that the client needs and will use.

➢ At the store, purchase items that do not need refrigeration first. Buy frozen items last.

➢ Be sure to read the label and review the unit pricing information on each item before you purchase it.

➢ When you return home, put away groceries immediately. Always put away frozen foods and items needing refrigeration first.

➢ Always remember to get a receipt for your purchases and return it to the client or the family along with the change.

CHAPTER 7

Storage and Handling of Food

Introduction

In this chapter, you will learn the safe way to handle food as you purchase it and as you store it in the refrigerator, the freezer, and the pantry. Since all food is not stored the same way and each food must be kept in the way best suited for the food and the method of storage, you must be familiar with the differences so that the food you prepare and the food that is eaten is always safe. You will also learn how to use the basic kitchen appliances and to safely prepare food for cooking.

Storage and handling of food is very important. It begins when the food is purchased. Once you purchase food, go directly home and put the refrigerated and frozen food items away first. If it is not possible to go directly home and the food will have to remain in a car or will be warm due to a long walk, think about the possibility of keeping the food cool either in a cooler or by packing some ice with the perishable food items. Items that are purchased prepared and ready to eat should be kept warm and eaten within two hours. Perishable foods should not be kept at room temperature longer that two hours. The harmful bacteria that cause food poisoning cannot be seen, smelled, or tasted. These bacteria multiply rapidly at room temperature. To avoid food poisoning it is extremely important to keep cold foods cold (40° F or below) and hot foods hot (above 140° F) (Figure 7.1) If your client does not have the ability to keep foods at their proper temperature, discuss this with your supervisor so a plan can be made to safely store food. Some people have a centigrade thermometer. Refer to Figure 7.2 for the way to work with both Fahrenheit and centigrade scales.

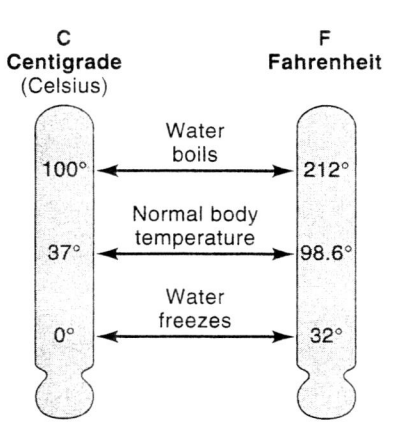

FIGURE 7.1 The two major scales for measuring temperature.

*H*ANDLING FOODS SAFELY

- Wash hands thoroughly in hot, soapy water *before* preparing foods and immediately *after* handling raw meat, poultry, or seafood.
- *Do not* let *raw juices* or *blood* from meats, poultry, or seafood touch ready-to-eat foods during preparation or when stored in the refrigerator. Keep hands, utensils, counters, cutting boards, and sinks clean. If using cutting boards, it is very important to keep them clean, especially if you use them for raw food products such as chicken and beef. Wash them in hot soapy water *immediately after* using them for chicken and beef and *before* using them for other food.
- *Do not* put cooked foods on the same plate that had raw meat or poultry on it.

*U*SING THE REFRIGERATOR SAFELY

- Keeping food in the refrigerator will preserve its freshness and keep it safe. The cold temperature will prevent the growth of most bacteria. This does not mean foods are safe indefinitely in the refrigerator. Food can spoil and **microorganisms** can still grow and multiply slowly over time, so there is a limit to the amount of time various foods will stay fresh in the refrigerator (Table 7.1).
- Set the refrigerator temperature at 40° F or below. Keep a refrigerator thermometer in the refrigerator and check the tempera-

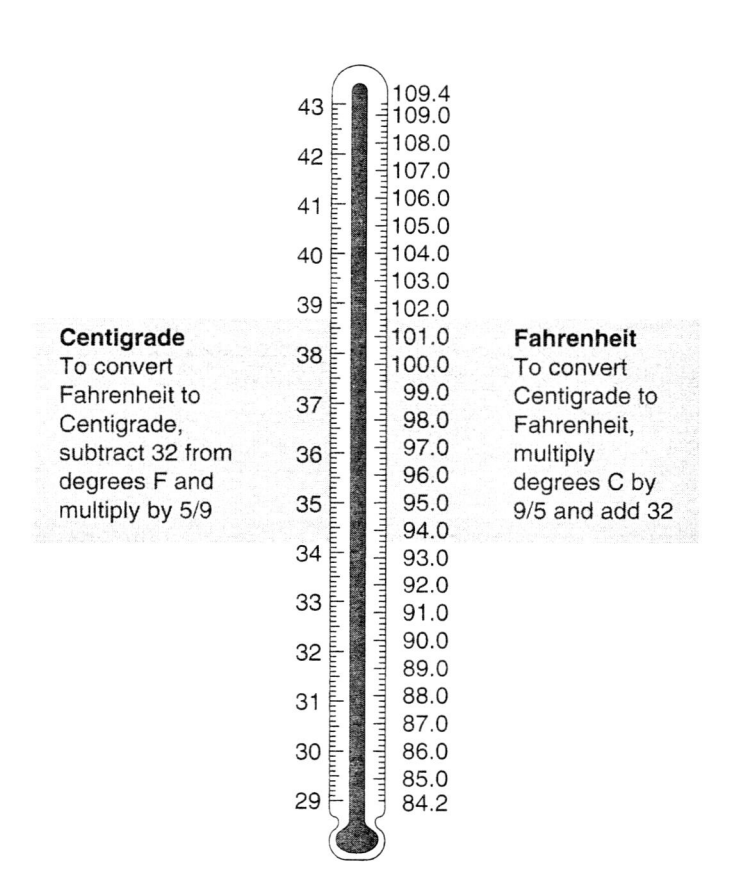

Centigrade
To convert Fahrenheit to Centigrade, subtract 32 from degrees F and multiply by 5/9

Fahrenheit
To convert Centigrade to Fahrenheit, multiply degrees C by 9/5 and add 32

FIGURE 7.2 Temperature conversion.

ture on a regular basis. The temperature of the refrigerator may need to be adjusted based on seasons, climate, and contents. A full refrigerator will require a lower temperature than an empty one. It is good idea to identify a suitable temperature setting and leave it. Air must be able to circulate freely to cool all foods evenly. Never pack a refrigerator so there is no room for air to circulate.

- Store foods in the refrigerator using airtight containers, foil, plastic wrap, or plastic bags that are leakproof. The correct method of storage will prevent foods from drying out and preserve freshness and appearance.
- Meat, fish, and poultry should be placed in the coldest part of the refrigerator, never in the door. Uncooked meats and poultry should be cooked or frozen within 1 to 2 days. Use or freeze cooked meats and poultry stored in the refrigerator within 3 to 4 days of their preparation.

Table 7.1 Guidelines for Safe Storage of Food Items

Food Item	Refrigerated	Frozen
Bananas—once ripened	2 days—skin will blacken	Whole peeled—1 month
Beef, pork, veal, lamb chops, steaks, roasts	3–5 days	4–12 months
Bread	7–14 days	3 months
Butter	1–3 months	6–9 months
Carrots	2 weeks	10–12 months
Chicken or turkey parts	1–2 days	9 months
Citrus fruits	1–2 weeks	Do not freeze
Cooked fish	3–4 days	4–6 months
Cottage cheese	1 week	Does not freeze well
Cream cheese	2 weeks	Does not freeze well
Cucumbers	4–5 days	Do not freeze
Deli meats—stored sliced	3–5 days	1–2 months
Eggs in shell	3–5 weeks	Do not freeze
Eggs substitutes, liquid, opened	3 days	Do not freeze
Eggs, hard cooked	1 week	Does not freeze well
Fish: cod, sole, haddock, flounder	1–2 days	6 months
Green beans	3–4 days	8 months
Ground chicken, turkey, or beef	1–2 days	3–4 months
Home-cooked meats	3–4 days	2–3 months
Milk	7 days	3 months
Mushrooms	2–3 days	10–12 months
Potatoes	1–2 weeks	Cooked, mashed, 10–12 months
Rolls	7 days	2 months
Spinach	1–2 days	10–12 months
Yogurt	7–14 days	1–2 months

- Eggs should be stored in their original container or another egg container, but not in the refrigerator door. Do not wash eggs before storing. This has been done in the commercial processing and is unnecessary. Never use cracked or dirty eggs.
- Defrost frozen foods in the refrigerator on a plate, not on the kitchen counter. They will become too warm on the counter and may spoil.
- Clean the refrigerator regularly to dispose of spoiled foods so bacteria will not pass to other foods in the refrigerator. Sweep regularly under the refrigerator so dust and crumbs do not accumulate.
- Do not leave the door of the refrigerator open for long periods of time so the temperature of the refrigerator does not get too warm.
- If the refrigerator is not a frost-free model, discuss with the client how it is defrosted.

Using the Freezer Safely

- Freezing food, either prepared or unprepared, is one way of keeping it safe for an extended period of time.
- Freeze food you do not plan to use or eat in a day or two. Frozen foods will taste better when defrosted if they were frozen at their peak quality time rather than at the end of their useful time.
- Proper packaging will prevent freezer burn and help foods maintain quality and taste. Many supermarket wrappings are air **permeable.** You may freeze in the original wrapper, but use the item within 1 to 2 months maximum. For items you wish to store longer, wrap with plastic wrap or heavy duty foil over the store wrap. You can also place the food item, still in the store wrap, in a plastic bag that is intended for freezer storage. Be sure to write on the wrapper the date, amount, and name of the item. Many items look the same in the freezer. By checking dates you will be able to use the oldest items first.
- If a food item does get **freezer burn,** it is still safe to consume. Freezer burn is a whitish area on the meat or poultry. It occurs when air touches the item and causes dry spots. This area can be cut away before or after cooking the food.

Using Microwave Ovens Safely

Microwave ovens are often used to defrost frozen food, cook food, or reheat foods. When using microwave ovens, remember that microwave heating can be uneven. Follow the microwave directions on the food label. Not all microwave ovens have the same power. Some foods easily become very hot and can splatter or explode if overheated. Regardless of how the container feels, the food may be a different temperature. The container may feel hot, but the food may not be hot. The container may feel cold, but the food can be very hot. Extreme caution must be used when using a microwave oven. Foods must be stirred thoroughly after heating to try to distribute the temperature evenly. The temperature of any foods or liquids heated in a microwave oven should be checked prior to giving it to any client in your care.

Defrosting Foods

Defrosting food requires some planning. It is important to maintain a safe, even temperature of the food while it is thawing. There are three safe ways to defrost food:

1. *In the refrigerator.* This is the longest method and may take several days depending on the size of the food. Place the food item on a plate or make sure it is tightly wrapped so that none the raw juices contaminate other foods in the refrigerator as the frozen item **thaws.**
2. *In cold water.* For a quick thaw, run *cold* water directly on the wrapped food item. This works particularly well for smaller items, such as a chicken breast. You may even place the item in cold water. Do not leave it for a prolonged period of time. The water can be emptied and replaced as often as necessary until the food is thawed. Never use hot water as this promotes bacteria growth.
3. *In the microwave.* Use the defrost feature, which uses less power than the cook feature. Remember to discuss this method with the family. Each microwave is different and has different power. This reduced power promotes even defrosting of both the outside of the item and the inside. If an item is not properly defrosted, the outside may be cooked and the inside still frozen. Microwave defrosting works well for ground items, such as ground beef. Food defrosted in the microwave should be cooked immediately after being defrosted.

Pantry Storage

- Items kept in the pantry must be safe at room temperature. Usually, these items should be kept in their original packaging so they remain sealed. A pantry should be located in a clean, dry, cool location and kept below 85° F. Storing in areas over 100° F or extreme cold can be dangerous and harmful for canned products. Never store foods in the pantry if the label states "keep refrigerated," even if you have not opened the item yet. You must read the package label to store the food item in the safest place. *Never use food from cans that are leaking, are badly dented, or have a foul odor when opened. Cracked jars or jars with loose or bulging lids should be avoided as well. Never taste or give to pets food items or from any container you are discarding.*

- Canned foods that are properly stored have a long shelf life. Most will remain safe to eat for several years.
- Canned poultry, meat, stews, soups (except tomato), potatoes, pasta products, corn, carrots, spinach, peas, beets, beans, and pumpkin will be safe for 2 years. These foods are considered low-acid food items.
- Tomato product, fruits, sauerkraut, and foods in vinegar-based dressings and sauces will be safe for up to 12 to 18 months.

DATING OF FOOD PRODUCTS

Dates are printed on many food products. There are many different types of dates:

- *Sell by.* This date tells the store how long to display the product for sale. This date represents the last day the product can be sold and still provides a reasonable period for home storage and consumption. Purchase the product *before* this date.
- *Best if used by.* This date tells the consumer when the food item will be at its best flavor and quality. It is not a purchase or safety date.
- *Use by.* This date tells the consumer the last date recommended for quality of the product. The date has been determined by the manufacturer of the food item.
- *Coded dates or numbers.* These are packing numbers used by manufacturers to track their products. This is the number used in the event of a recall. Manufacturers also use this number in determining how to rotate their stock and what to ship to the distribution warehouses.

TIPS FOR COOKING SAFELY

- Cook crumbled ground meats until all pink color is gone and the juices run clear, not red or pink. The center of patties and meat loaf are safe when the internal temperature reaches 160° F; ground poultry patties and loaves should reach 165° F.

- Rinse seafood and poultry in cold, running water before cooking.
- **Marinate** vegetables, meats, fish, or poultry in self-closing plastic bags or in covered containers. Always marinate foods in the refrigerator, never on the countertop. Do not add liquid used for marinating to food items once food has started to cook. The raw juices in the marinade may not have adequate time to cook. If you want to use or serve the extra liquid, bring the marinated juices to a boil and maintain for at least 1 minute to help kill any bacteria that could be in the juices from the raw product.
- When grilling, broiling, or roasting, use different plates for the raw and cooked products. Using the same plate can cause **cross-contamination**.
- During grilling, broiling, or cooking on the stove, turn meats over at least once.
- When baking, do not set the oven temperature lower than 325° F unless the recipe specifically calls for you to do so. When using the microwave oven, cover meats with plastic wrap, and halfway through the cooking process, rotate the dish and turn the meat item over. Ground meats should be stirred once or twice. Microwaved meats should stand before eating to complete the cooking process. Use a meat thermometer to check several spots as the temperatures in the various sections of the meat will vary. The amount of time the meat should stand will vary depending on how large the item is and how long it cooked. It most likely will be between 5 minutes and 30 minutes.
- To reheat leftovers, cover and heat, by the method you choose, until at least 165° F or hot and steaming throughout.

YOUR ROLE AS A HOMEMAKER/HOME HEALTH AIDE

Helping clients store their food is a big responsibility. The way you do it will affect the ease and safety with which they can get the food when you are not in the home. Try and be sensitive to the way that the client keeps his food. Be sure, however, that the food is stored properly and safely. If you notice that it is not, discuss this with your client. If a change is not able to be made, alert the family and your supervisor. Sometimes a change is not welcome because it will result in additional expense. Sometimes a change is not welcome because the client is unfamiliar with the practice. If the change is needed because of safety and it is not welcome, be sure to report this.

POINTS TO REMEMBER

➤ Handwashing is the single most important activity to prevent illness and keep a clean kitchen.
➤ Keep all utensils clean and wash them after using them with meat, fish, and poultry and before using them with other food.
➤ Store food in the correct place. Keep perishable food cool in a refrigerator or cooler until ready to use.
➤ Food kept in a pantry or freezer cannot be kept indefinitely. Check dates for safe use.
➤ Never taste or use food from a can if it is bulging, leaking, or has a foul odor when opened.
➤ The danger zone for rapid growth of bacteria is 40° F to 140° F.
➤ Discuss the use of the appliances with the family. Every appliance is somewhat different. Do not assume they are all alike.

Meat - brownish grey.
Poultry - juice clear
fish - big flakes

CHAPTER 8
Sodium-Restricted Diet

Introduction

This chapter will familiarize you with the many ways the body uses salt to maintain itself. Salt, or sodium, can be either helpful or harmful to the body. You will learn basic ways to help maintain the sodium level that is appropriate for your client by assisting with the choice and preparation of foods.

Salt is one of the nutrients the human body needs to live. Salt has been used as money, as an agent to preserve foods, as a medication, and as a substance to enhance the taste of food. Sodium is part of salt. The other part of salt is chloride. Sodium also is found in food, water, and plants. The amount of salt and the effect it has on our bodies varies from person to person and from season to season. The words sodium and salt are often used interchangeably, but they are not the same. Salt is only one source of sodium.

WHY THE BODY NEEDS SODIUM

The human body has several different types of fluids in it. The amount of sodium in the body is one of the factors that determine the amounts of the various fluids. Sodium works with potassium, another mineral, to maintain the balance of fluids. When one of these nutrients is out of balance with the other or with the body in general, the amount of fluid is affected. Sodium is also necessary for the transportation of **glucose** and other nutrients in and out of all bodily cells, for muscle contraction, and for the transmission of electrical nerve impulses in the body.

SODIUM LEVELS IN THE BODY

The correct level of sodium in the body is obtained by balancing the sodium retention and sodium loss. When this balance is upset due to disease, medication, or dietary changes, the body is affected. Sodium levels are different for different people. Levels of activity, the way the body processes the sodium, and the state of a person's health all determine the appropriate sodium level. A health care professional will examine the client; take into consideration his total health, age, and the medication he is taking; and prescribe a diet that indicates the amount of sodium that should be eaten during a 24-hour period. Sometimes the amount of sodium will be restricted and sometimes it will not.

- The need for sodium changes with age and should be adjusted accordingly. The physician will determine changes as needed.
- There is a unique relationship of sodium and certain cardiovascular and kidney diseases. The levels of sodium intake is always prescribed by a health care professional and should not be changed without consulting one who has the entire medical history and medication schedule available.
- The level of sodium intake during pregnancy is determined by the client's physician and varies from client to client.

MAINTAINING A SODIUM-RESTRICTED DIET

A sodium-restricted diet should be treated as you would treat any prescribed medication. After all, when changing the sodium content of the diet, the whole functioning of the body is changed as it would be with any prescribed medication. The amount of sodium that should be eaten by your client will be prescribed in **milligrams.** A low-sodium diet, limiting the amount of sodium in the diet to 2,000 mg, is most commonly ordered. This amount is about half of the sodium in an average diet.

Sodium free	Contains 5 milligrams or less of sodium per serving
Very low sodium	35 milligrams or less of sodium per serving
Low sodium	140 milligrams or less of sodium per serving
Reduced sodium	At least 25% less sodium than the original version, but be cautious—this product may still contain a significant amount of sodium
No added salt or unsalted	No salt is added during processing, but this does not mean it is sodium free

When purchasing food, it is important to understand the labeling terminology. It is the key to understanding what is meant when a product's sodium content has been reduced.

One teaspoon of table salt (sodium chloride) contains approximately 2,000 mg of sodium. This is the most common restriction.

The Impact of a Sodium-Restricted Diet

Often, changing the amount of sodium may mean big changes in cooking and eating favorite or ethnically familiar foods. Some families find it hard to change their cooking habits for one member of the family. This can cause problems in the kitchen, at the table, and with family dynamics. Your role will be to help the client maintain his or her diet while still having a balanced diet that is enjoyable and acceptable to the family. A family may decide to cook without salt and let everyone add salt to their tastes at the table, or they may decide to cook your client's food separately. By working with the family and the client a suitable plan can be established. If, however, you find that you cannot establish a plan that meets the client's needs and the family's needs, discuss this with your supervisor.

Helpful Hints

- Read food labels carefully. Anything that contains the word *sodium* has some sodium in it. Look at the amount of sodium on the label.
- Rinse canned foods such as canned vegetables or tuna to remove the salty juices or buy them packed in water.
- If foods have been packed in **brine,** rinse them well before using.
- *Do not* add salt to your foods when cooking or at the table before eating.
- Start to cook foods from scratch using low-sodium ingredients.
- Use herbs, spices, and fruit juices to season food.
- Limit the amount of highly processed or prepared foods you buy and consume.
- Read the label of condiments and spices such as ketchup, mustard, and steak sauce.
- Avoid fast foods, which are very high in salt, as are many restaurant foods.
- Request that food in a restaurant be prepared without salt.
- If meat is salted before cooking for religious reasons, as with kosher meat, discuss with the health care professional which substitute products may be used.

The following list includes foods high in sodium that should *not* be included in your daily diet if you are trying to limit your daily amount of sodium intake.

A-1 sauce	Anchovies	Bacon	Barbecue sauce
Bologna	Bouillon cubes or powders (regular)	Buttermilk	Canned gravies or sauces
Canned ravioli or spaghetti	Canned soups	Canned stews	Canned vegetables
Catsup	Caviar	Celery salt	Cheese doodles
Chili sauce	Corned beef	Cheese—regular, processed, and spreads	Chinese food, canned or restaurant
Frozen breaded meats and fish	Frozen TV dinners	Ham—smoked or cured	Hamburger Helper mix
Herring	Horseradish	Hot dogs/ frankfurters	Kitchen Bouquet
Knockwurst	Kosher meats	Liverwurst	Lox
Luncheon meats	Malted milk	Meat tenderizers	Monosodium glutamate (Accent)
Mustard	Nuts—salted	Olives	Onion salt
Party spread and dips	Pastrami	Pickled pigs feet	Pickles
Popcorn— salted	Relishes	Salami	Salted snack foods—pretzels, potato chips, corn chips
Sardines	Sausage	Sauerkraut	Scrapple
Sea salt	Seasoned salt	Smoked salmon	Smoked tongue
Soy sauce	Tomato juice— regular	Worcestershire sauce	

Using Herbs and Spices

You can prepare foods that taste good with less salt and sodium by using herbs and spices. Herbs also add color and interest to the food. Herbs and spices can add and enhance flavors of all foods. They are low in sodium or sodium free and fat free. Common spices to have on hand when trying to limit sodium intake include:

- Basil
- Bay leaf
- Chili powder
- Cinnamon
- Dry mustard
- Garlic powder (*not* garlic salt)
- Ginger
- Onion powder (*not* onion salt)
- Oregano
- Paprika
- Parsley
- Pepper, black ground
- Pepper, red crushed
- Thyme
- Various blends (*not* salt seasoning blends)

Most salt substitutes contain potassium for flavor, which may not be appropriate for all clients. Check with the health care professional who prescribed the sodium-restricted diet as to which salt substitute is permitted.

Your Role as a Homemaker/Home Health Aide

As clients learn to change their use of salt, they will need your encouragement and suggestions. Be alert to point out positive changes and continue to make creative suggestions so that clients can meet their goals. Your help and suggestions to the family will be very important. Sometimes, family members are not aware that their actions or comments are not supporting your client's needs. If a client doesn't eat properly one day, try to find out the reason and encourage him or her to return to the plan. Do not scold clients or make them feel that they have failed. Discuss with your supervisor ways you could help them get back to the plan.

POINTS TO REMEMBER

➤ Salt is necessary for the body to function properly. The level that each person needs may differ.

➤ A sodium-restricted diet is prescribed by a physician and should be treated as you would treat any prescribed medication.

➤ Reading labels on cans, boxes of foods, and over-the-counter medications is one the most important things you can do to identify foods that contain added sodium.

➤ Using herbs and spices will flavor food so that the sodium is not missed.

CHAPTER 9

Fat- and Cholesterol-Restricted Diets

Introduction

Healthy eating is what fat- and cholesterol-restricted diets are all about. An abundant amount of choices are available to us today. New information is continually being presented about the role fat and cholesterol play in maintaining health. Although the amount of fat in each diet must be individually prescribed, each individual is affected differently by these substances, and doctors and health care professionals have differing views, there are certain basic facts that are not disputed. Changing the amount of fat in one's diet should be done with the supervision of a qualified health practitioner. The effect should be monitored over time. In this chapter, you will become familiar with the types of fat present in food and in the body. You will also learn some basic ways to help your clients change the amount of fat in their diet through wise meal planning and careful cooking. Changing the amount of fat in a diet is a process that takes careful supervision from the health care professional and those who do the cooking and the food purchasing.

Fats

The word **lipid** is used to identify fats that are found in the bloodstream. **Body fat** is a term used to identify the fat that is stored in the body and available after it is converted to usable energy. **Dietary lipids** are fats that are ingested rather than fat that the body manufactures. A moderate amount of both types of fat is necessary for the body to function properly. It is important to know the difference between fat that is beneficial and fat that is potentially harmful.

- Fat is necessary for the absorption of the fat-soluble vitamins and to maintain skin integrity.
- Fats gives flavor to food and increase our enjoyment of food.
- Body fat assists with regulating and maintaining the temperature of the body.
- Body fat helps protect organs and internal tissues.
- Body fat assists with hormone production, storage, and regulation.

Fat is a major energy source for the body, but it is not the only source of energy. Too much fat can be harmful to the body, especially the circulatory system, as it raises blood **cholesterol levels.** Increased blood cholesterol levels are associated with heart attacks and strokes. Americans have slowly increased their consumption of fats over time. This phenomenon and the fact that research has identified the long-term effects of high fat consumption on the human body have led to the present awareness that too much fat is not healthy.

All types of fats contain the same 9 calories per gram. Therefore, changing the type of fat will not alter the caloric intake. Since a certain amount of fat is necessary for proper cell function and skin integrity, it is important to balance the intake of fat with the appropriate caloric intake.

Fat and cholesterol are not the same. If a client is advised to decrease cholesterol intake, the diet may not be the same as it is for the client who is advised to decrease fat intake. Keep this in mind when planning meals, reading food labels, and monitoring food intake.

Sources of Fat

Small amounts of fat are present in almost all food we eat. The fat may be visible or invisible. The main sources of fats are:

- Meat, poultry, fish
- Oils, both solid and liquid
- Nuts
- Sauces and spreads
- Dairy products such as cheese, milk, and butter
- Certain vegetables such as avocados, olives, and soybeans

Types of Fats

There are many types of fats and many fatty acids. Facts about them are being discovered all the time. The best rule is to discuss with a nutritionist choices of margarine, oils, and foods high in fats so the diet can be individualized for your client.

- *Saturated fats* tend to be hard. They are solid at room temperature. They interfere with the removal of cholesterol from the bloodstream. They are found mainly in meats and dairy products made with whole milk. Some vegetables oils, such as palm oil and coconut oil, and cocoa butter act like saturated fats and should be avoided.
- *Hydrogenated* vegetable oils should be avoided. Hydrogenation involves a manufacturing procedure that adds hydrogen to the vegetable oil, making it solid at room temperature. Hydrogenated vegetable oils are saturated fats even though they were once vegetable oils.
- *Polyunsaturated fats* are liquid at room temperature. Sunflower, safflower, corn, soybean, cottonseed, and sesame oils are all polyunsaturated.
- *Monounsaturated fats* are liquid at room temperature, semisolid or solid when refrigerated. Olive, peanut, and canola oils are examples of monounsaturated fats. These may help lower cholesterol levels in the blood.

CHOLESTEROL

Cholesterol is a waxy substance found in foods of animal origin. It is also manufactured by the body in the liver. You need only very small amounts. This type of fat, both in the bloodstream and stored in the body, has been identified as a high-risk factor when discussing heart conditions, high blood pressure, and certain types of cancers. Although it is only one risk factor, it is important to remember that we now know many ways of decreasing and/or controlling cholesterol.

Although we ingest fats in many forms, cholesterol is one fat that we both ingest and is produced by the human body in the liver.

- *VLDL (very low-density lipoprotein)* (consists primarily of triglycerides) carries fats to different parts of the body
- *LDL (low-density lipoprotein)* carries cholesterol to different parts of the body; "bad" cholesterol because it may become stuck in the blood vessels and block the blood flow causing a clot, high blood pressure, or disease. The lower this number, the better.
- *HDL (high-density lipoprotein)* carries cholesterol left in the bloodstream to the liver; "good" cholesterol because it brings cholesterol to the liver and helps remove it from the blood vessels and bloodstream. The higher this number, the better. Exercise as well as dietary modifications can help raise this level in the blood.

Reducing Cholesterol

When a person has been advised to reduce his or her cholesterol intake, it is usually part of an entire health promotion regime. Although a change in diet is very important, all of the following activities contribute to the overall reduction in cholesterol:

- Stop smoking.
- Increase exercise.
- Watch total caloric intake, modifying it to lose weight or gain weight.
- Increase dietary fiber, which decreases the absorption of cholesterol.
- Decrease dietary fat intake, focusing on lowering cholesterol intake.
- Drink alcohol in moderation.
- Take medication as prescribed.
- Read labels and focus on purchasing, preparing, and eating low-fat items.

The National Cholesterol Education Program advocates a stepwise approach to reduce serum lipids.

Step 1 Diet The step 1 diet is the first level of treatment for those with high blood cholesterol in many adults and children over the age of two. It is similar to the recommendation for the general population.

Step 2 Diet The step 2 diet is much more restrictive and used following the step 1 diet when no improvements are seen after 8 to 12 weeks. It is also used when evidence of fatty deposits in the arteries is known or a heart attack or stroke has already occurred.

	Step 1 Diet	Step 2 Diet
Total Fat	No more than 30% of total calories	No more than 30% of total calories
Saturated Fat	8–10% of total fat calories from saturated fats	Less than 7% of the total fat calories from saturated fats
Cholesterol	No more than 300 mg/day	No more than 200 mg/day
Meats and protein sources	Limit to 6 ounces daily	Limit to 5 ounces daily
Eggs	Limit to 4 egg yolks per week	Limit to 1 egg yolk per week

Changing Cooking Habits

Changing cooking habits and food preference is a difficult task. It often involves cooking differently for one person in the family. It also means that favorite foods, ethnically based foods, and often inexpensive foods can no longer be eaten in the same quantities.

- Do not add fats to foods as you grill, roast, microwave, or steam them but rather use nonstick sprays to prevent sticking and add flavor.
- Remove all visible fat from food before cooking.
- Use herbs and spices for seasoning.
- Use light or nonfat spreads.
- Decrease meat intake and increase use of fish, poultry, and legumes.
- Use vegetable oil in place of lard, butter, or margarine.
- Decrease use of eggs by using egg substitutes.
- Reduce portion size.
- Snack on low-fat pretzels, popcorn, vegetables, crackers, or fruit.
- Eliminate fried foods.
- Eliminate prepared foods.
- Eliminate fast foods.

Common Recipe Substitutions

1 egg yolk	1 egg white or $\frac{1}{8}$ cup egg substitute
1 whole egg	2 egg whites or $\frac{1}{4}$ cup egg substitute
Whole milk products	Skim milk products if available
Cream	Evaporated skim milk
Butter or shortening	Oils or margarine that are monounsaturated or polyunsaturated fats
Sour cream	Skim milk yogurt

Olestra

Olestra is a calorie-free fat substitute. It is used in the place of regular cooking oils or other fats. It gives the same texture to the food and feel in your mouth as if it were a regular fat. Olestra is processed from vegetable oil and sugar. It cannot be absorbed by the body and therefore passes through the body unchanged and does not provide calories. When ingesting foods containing Olestra, your body may not efficiently absorb vitamins A, D, E, and K. Currently, foods containing Olestra also contain these vitamins. Carbohydrates, proteins, fats, minerals, and water-soluble vitamins are not affected by Olestra. When reading food labels, Olestra may appear as Olean. Remember, the best way to reduce fat in your diet is to limit the total amount of fat ingested. Also be careful of portion sizes, and include physical activity if possible.

YOUR ROLE AS A HOMEMAKER/HOME HEALTH AIDE

Reducing the amount of fat or changing the fat used in cooking often requires great effort. Cultural practices may have to be changed. Tastes may have to be altered. If all members of the family do not wish to make the change, your client may have to either cook separately, eat separately, or not make the recommended change. Either way, your support and understanding will be essential.

- All fats in the diet must be reduced, but it is especially important to avoid saturated fats.
- Read all food labels if you are responsible for shopping or food preparation.
- Report to your supervisor compliance and noncompliance of the client in your care.

POINTS TO REMEMBER

➤ Fat is necessary in a balanced diet to promote a healthy body. Elimination of all fat will not permit the digestion of fat-soluble vitamins, healthy skin, or healthy cell metabolism.
➤ The decrease of dietary cholesterol is part of a whole regime usually associated with exercise, a change in food preparation, and possibly medication.
➤ Support the client who is changing a lifetime food habit.

CHAPTER 10

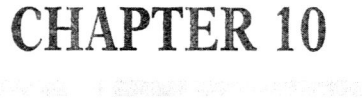

Diabetic Diets

Introduction

In this chapter, you will become familiar with the types of diabetes and the ways in which people alter their diet to live with this chronic disease. Your role in assisting the client and the family to become comfortable with the changes and with incorporating the dietary needs of the client into daily life is an important part of the client's acceptance of his disease.

Diabetes mellitus, or diabetes, is the most common disease of the **endocrine** system. The millions of people who have this chronic disease are unable to break down the food they eat into usable glucose to produce energy and cell growth. This chronic condition is a result of the body's inability to produce and regulate the hormone **insulin.** People who have this disease do not outgrow it, but have it to one degree or another all their lives. If the disease is managed with proper diet, exercise, and sometimes medication, people can lead normal, productive, long lives. If however, diet, medication, and exercise regimes are not maintained, complications to all body systems and organs can occur. Diet is the most important treatment for those with diabetes. (See Table 10.1 for the three forms of diabetes.)

WHO IS AT RISK FOR DIABETES?

Although the cause of diabetes is not yet known, risk factors are generally accepted as:

- Obesity, especially those who are more than 140% of their desirable body weight and/or whose excess weight is distributed in their upper part of their body

Table 10.1 Three Forms of Diabetes

Type	Characteristics	Treatment
Type 1: Insulin-dependent diabetes mellitus (IDDM) (juvenile diabetes)	Onset usually before age 30 but can develop at any age; person cannot make the hormone insulin; person usually within weight guidelines or underweight, sometimes weight loss has occurred before diagnosis.	Diet, exercise, insulin injections
Type 2: Non–insulin-dependent diabetes mellitus (NIDDM) (adult-onset diabetes)	Most common form, usually develops gradually after age 40; insulin production may be decreased, increased, or normal, but the body is unable to utilize it; person usually overweight, may have high blood pressure, or a family history of diabetes.	Diet, exercise, weight control; may take oral hypoglycemics
Gestational diabetes	Develops only during pregnancy; overweight and/or older women are more susceptible.	Diet, insulin may be prescribed. Usually disappears after pregnancy but, Type 1 or 2 may appear later in life.

- Family history
- Presence of hypertension
- Presence of high cholesterol
- Being over 45 years old
- Having delivered a baby over 9 pounds with or without the presence of gestational diabetes
- Being African American, Hispanic, or Native American

SIGNS AND SYMPTOMS OF DIABETES MELLITUS

- Fatigue
- Loss of weight
- Sores that heal slowly
- High blood sugar

- Frequent and large amounts of urine
- Excessive thirst
- Poor vision
- Inflammation of the vagina

THE IMPORTANCE OF MAINTAINING A DIABETIC DIET

For your clients, identifying and following their individualized prescribed diet is as important as taking medication in its prescribed manner. For people with diabetes, food helps control their diabetes by controlling the level of glucose in their blood. Therefore, food and the timing of meals, with or without medication, must be viewed as the treatment for the disease and treated with great importance.

Careful meal planning plays a significant role in managing diabetes. Good nutritional principles include eating a variety of different foods, balancing food choices from the Food Pyramid, and keeping all nutrients to a prescribed level rather than overeating on one food item. Focus on foods low in fat and high in complex carbohydrates and fiber. Keep blood glucose, blood lipid levels, and individual weight goals in mind as you make food choices. Balancing the diabetic needs of the client with other medical conditions can be a challenge. For instances, some diabetic clients must also maintain a low-sodium diet. Others may have to limit their fat, cholesterol, or calorie intake. Remember to keep all these client needs in mind when you plan meals, purchase food, and prepare meals. It is extremely important that meal plans be realistic and based on the client's food preferences and the type of insulin prescribed. If insulin is administered, it is critical to have food distributed so it interacts with the timing of the insulin in the body. Some prescribed meal plans may indicate that the client should eat three meals and a bedtime snack, others five or six small meals and a bedtime snack. Your client should have clear guidelines for you to follow. Exchange lists are used very often as a guideline for food selection and portion amounts. If your client does not have a specific dietary plan, discuss this with your supervisor immediately so that you can determine what specific dietary requirements exist. Refer to Chapter 3 for things to take into account when planning your client's meals.

GUIDELINES TO MAINTAINING A DIABETIC DIET

Guidelines for maintaining a diabetic diet are very similar to guidelines for maintaining a regular, healthy diet. They take into account the client's general health, medication, and particular likes and dislikes. The following are general guidelines and may be changed by the client's health care professional if there is a documented reason. Diabetics, however, must always be aware of the timing and the dosage of their medication in relation to their meals.

- Caloric needs are based on maintaining a healthy weight. If weight loss is desired, then calories may be reduce to promote weight loss.
- Protein should be about 10 to 20 percent of total calories in the form of both animal and vegetable protein.
- Fat intake should be limited to no more than 30 percent of total calories. Saturated fat should be limited to 10 percent or less. Dietary cholesterol intake should be limited to 300 mg or less per day.
- Carbohydrate intake is usually measured in total carbohydrate rather than specific sources. Carbohydrates are distributed along with protein and fat throughout the meal plan in the forms of meals and snacks.
- Fiber, especially water-soluble fiber, is recommended to help regulate and maintain stable blood glucose levels. The recommendations at this time are between 20 and 35 grams per day.

Eating in a Restaurant

Restaurant foods can be incorporated into a diabetic regimen. All the guidelines that are followed at home are adaptable to dining out. All food choices should be carefully made. Portion sizes must be maintained, and excess food may be brought home for consumption at a later time. It is important not to overeat in a restaurant just because the food has been paid for. Blood glucose levels should be maintained whether clients are preparing their own food or eating out. Discussion with the waiter as to how food is prepared and portion size should take place before the food is brought to the table.

Signs and Symptoms of Diabetic Coma *hyperglycemia*

Diabetic coma occurs when the blood has too many carbohydrates and not enough insulin to metabolize them. The symptoms include:

- Heavy, labored breathing and increased respirations
- Loss of appetite
- Dulled senses
- Nausea and/or vomiting
- Weakness

- Abdominal pain or discomfort
- Generalized aches
- Increased thirst or parched tongue
- Sweet or fruity-smelling breath
- Flushed, dry skin
- Increased urination
- Soft eyeballs
- On examination, large amounts of sugar in the urine and high blood sugar

SIGNS AND SYMPTOMS OF INSULIN SHOCK hypoGlycemia

Insulin shock occurs when a person's blood has more insulin that the amount of carbohydrates available for metabolism. The symptoms include:

- Excessive sweating, perspiration
- Faintness, dizziness, weakness
- Hunger
- Irritability, personality changes, nervousness
- Numbness of tongue or lips
- Inability to awaken, coma, unconsciousness, stupor
- Headache
- Tremors, trembling
- Blurred or impaired vision
- On examination, low blood sugar and no sugar in the urine

YOUR ROLE AS A HOMEMAKER/HOME HEALTH AIDE

It is important that you understand what diabetes is and how to help your client and his or her family live with this chronic disease. Prescribed food and medication regimes should be followed and not changed without physician input. Understanding how food, medication, and activity contribute to blood glucose levels and learning to maintain appropriate blood glucose levels within the recommended guidelines is important. If your client does not have a clear understanding of the disease; the interaction of food, exercise, and medication; and the results of straying from the prescribed regimen, discuss this with your supervisor so that additional information and teaching can be scheduled. *If your client exhibits any symptoms of insulin food imbalance, it is essential that you call your supervisor or follow the emergency procedure established in the home.*

Medication should be stored in a convenient place away from children. If the client does not remember the times that medication should be taken, write them down. If the client does not remember if medication was taken, create a method for the client to document each dose. Insulin should be kept in a cool place, away from heat and strong light. Sometimes it is kept in the refrigerator. Keep syringes in a safe place and dispose of them the way your supervisor suggests so that local ordinances regarding regulated medical waste are met.

If you notice that your client does not adhere to his medication or eating schedule, notify your supervisor immediately. Diets can be changed or tailored to individual needs. For instance, children may obtain their calories from different foods than the elderly do. People without teeth may need different foods than those who are able to chew.

It is critical to the client not to administer insulin or take oral hypoglycemics unless mealtimes are maintained. Insulin doses are usually based on caloric intake, meal plans, and blood glucose levels.

You may be asked to assist clients as they test their blood glucose levels before or after meals. If clients are able to perform this themselves, they should continue this when you are in the house. Be sure that you are aware of how this blood check is continued when you are not in the house. Discuss with your supervisor when you should report blood glucose levels and to whom they should be reported.

POINTS TO REMEMBER

➤ Diabetes is a chronic disease that can be controlled through prescribed food, exercise, and medication.

➤ Noncompliance to the prescribed regimen should be reported to your supervisor immediately so that adjustments in the medication or caloric intake can also be made.

➤ Diabetic diets are prescribed just as medication is prescribed and individualized. Changes can be made only by a physician.

➤ Diabetic management is a continually changing effort. Assist clients as they note bodily changes as well as changes in reaction to their medication, diet, and exercise level.

CHAPTER 11

Additional Dietary Considerations and Modifications

Introduction

In this chapter you will learn some of the ways in which diets may be modified to meet a client's needs. These needs may be temporary or permanent, and the **modifications** may last for a few days or for years. The modifications include adding **fiber,** changing the consistency of the food, or eliminating one food product due to allergy or intolerance. When this is done, it must be done with the whole client, his medication, his culture, and his unique needs taken into consideration. Although there seem to be dietary fads, changes should be made only in consultation with a health care practitioner who is able to view the total nutrition and the total health of the client. Do not change diets in response to articles in the newspaper or guests on a TV talk show.

DIETARY FIBER

Dietary fiber is important in a healthy diet for all ages. Fiber is found only in plants such as vegetables, fruits, and grains (Table 11.1). The part of the plant fiber that is eaten is called **dietary fiber.**

Table 11.1 Some Common Sources of Fiber

Food	Serving Size	Total Fiber (in grams)	Soluble Fiber (in grams)	Insoluble Fiber (in grams)
Apple with skin	1 medium	3.0	0.5	2.5
Banana	1 medium	2.0	0.5	1.5
Bran flake cereal	3/4 cup	5.5	0.5	5.0
Broccoli	1/2 cup	2.0	0	2.0
Corn	1/2 cup	1.5	0	1.5
Kidney beans	1/2 cup	4.5	1.0	3.5
Oatmeal—cooked	3/4 cup	3.0	1.0	2.0
Orange	1 medium	2.0	0.5	1.5
Spinach	1/2 cup	2.0	0.5	1.5
Whole-wheat bread	1 slice	2.5	0.5	2.0

Dietary fiber consists of soluble and insoluble fiber. **Soluble fiber** forms a gel in the digestive tract, while insoluble fiber does not. **Insoluble fiber** passes through the digestive tract unchanged. Both fibers are important and provide benefits to a healthy digestive system by maintaining regularity of bowel movements.

Soluble fiber offers help in controlling blood cholesterol levels by binding to some cholesterol in the digestive tract and removing it from the body naturally. Soluble fiber is found in:

- Oats
- Peas
- Some fruits, such as banana
- Psyllium (grain found in some cereals, dietary supplements, and fiber laxatives)

The current recommendation for an average adult is to eat 20 to 35 grams of soluble and insoluble fiber each day. Children should eat 5 grams/day plus their age. For example, a 10 year old should eat 10 + 5 = 15 grams per day.

The average American eats about 12 to 17 grams of fiber a day due to the increased use of refined grains and fast foods.

Adding Fiber to a Diet

The decision to add fiber to a diet should be made by the health care professional, the client, and the family. Since adding fiber affects the digestive system, it is important to view the entire dietary intake of a person when making this decision. Fiber can be added through powders and tablets when necessary, but getting it through foods should be tried first unless instructed otherwise by a health care professional. When adding fiber:

- Add in small increments to the diet. Let the body get used to the change before adding more.
- Drink at least 8 glasses of water a day.
- Discuss the effect additional fiber may have on medication and vitamin absorption with your supervisor.
- Monitor the effect of the additional fiber on bowel movements, gas, and reaction to medication.

Low-Residue or Low-Fiber Diet

In some instances, a chronic or acute medical condition would indicate the need to **restrict** fiber. These diseases include but are not limited to acute phases of diverticulitis, Crohn's disease, or ulcerative colitis. Occasionally after intestinal surgery, including colostomy or ileostomy placement, a **low-residue, low-fiber diet** is recommended for a short period of time (Table 11.2).

If this diet is followed for a prolonged period of time, the intake of fruits and vegetables may not be adequate. On a low-residue diet the intake of calcium may need to be monitored. A multivitamin may be needed, or additional liquid supplements may be prescribed by the health care professional.

Clear Liquid Diet

The **clear liquid diet** includes beverages that are both clear and liquid at body temperature. This diet helps to relieve thirst, helps to maintain fluid and electrolyte balance, and helps stimulate **peristalsis** after surgery. Because of the limited choices, this diet is inadequate for most nutrients and should be followed only for a day or so. If needed longer, a nutritional evaluation in consultation with the client's physician should be done to ensure adequate nutrition.

Table 11.2 Low-Residue or Low-Fiber Diet Recommendations

Group	Foods Recommended	Foods to Avoid
Milk and milk products (limit to 2 cups daily)	All milk products okay	Only 2 cups daily of all milk products
Starches—bread and grains	All bread and cereals made from refined flours, pasta, white rice	Whole-grain breads, cereals, rice, pasta, bran cereals, oatmeal
Vegetables	Lettuce; only the following cooked: yellow squash without seeds, green beans, wax beans, spinach, pumpkin, eggplant, potatoes without skin, asparagus, beets, carrots	Vegetables juices with pulp, raw vegetables except lettuce, all other cooked vegetables not previously listed
Fruits	All canned fruit except pineapple, ripe bananas, melons, fruit juices without pulp	Fruit juices with pulp, canned pineapple, prunes, prune juice, dried fruit, jam, marmalade, fresh fruits except ripe banana, and melons
Meats and substitutes	Meat, poultry, eggs, and seafood	Chunky peanut butter, nuts, seeds, dried beans, peas
Fats and oils	All oils, margarine, and butter	Coconut
Miscellaneous		Popcorn, pickles, horseradish, relish, foods containing nuts and coconut

- Foods included are tea, coffee, fat-free broth, ginger ale, clear fruit juices, fruit ices, and plain-flavored gelatins.
- *No* milk or milk products.
- Oral supplements may be included as directed by the health care professional, if they are considered clear liquids.

FULL LIQUID DIET

The **full liquid diet** includes foods that liquefy at body temperature. This diet can be nutritionally adequate. It is high in fat and calcium and low in fiber. Protein in the diet can be increased by adding nonfat dry milk to milk-based food items. This diet is usually very high in **lactose,** which is inappropriate for those on lactose restriction.

Foods included are:

- Milk and all milk products
- Cooked thin cereal, strained soups, and all juices
- All foods allowed on a clear liquid diet
- Fiber (may have to be added as a supplement)

SOFT DIET

A **soft diet** consists of foods that are easily digestible, usually low in fiber, soft in consistency, and **bland** in flavor. It can be used as a transitional period before a "regular" meal plan is followed, although some people remain on this diet for extended periods of time. Since the main difference between a soft diet and a regular diet is the selection of foods and the lack of spice, it is usually nutritionally adequate. The consistencies of the food items *do not* have to be altered. *Soft* refers to soft to the digestive tract.

MECHANICAL SOFT DIET

The **mechanical soft diet** is appropriate for those who have difficulty in chewing. Sometimes this is due to poor-fitting dentures or no teeth at all. It is also used for those who have had a stroke or neck or head surgery. The only change from the "normal" or "regular" diet is the texture. There is no restriction on seasoning or methods of food preparation. This diet should not be overly restricted. Clients' ability to chew will vary greatly. Careful evaluation and observation during mealtimes is necessary.

Common modifications to provide mechanical soft foods include:

- Vegetables are well cooked. They can even be minced or diced if necessary.
- Soft raw fruits like banana, berries, citrus sections; melons can be partially mashed. All cooked canned and frozen fruits can be included.
- Meat and poultry are ground or minced. Fish is usually tender enough and does not need further mincing.
- Bread should be soft, including rolls and biscuits, instead of crisp and crusty.
- All dessert allowed on "normal/regular" diet that are soft, such as pudding, custards, cakes, and some pies.

PUREED DIET

The **pureed diet** includes foods that are smooth and soft. These foods are easy to swallow and require little or no chewing. All foods are

blenderized and pureed unless already smooth. If a blender is not available, put the food through a food mill or a sieve. Liquids, such as soup, can be added to create a consistency appropriate for each client. Commercial products are available to change the consistency of foods.

- Do not offer baby food to adults, unless instructed, as baby foods will not meet the nutritional needs of adults.
- To increase intake and make the plate look more attractive, puree each food item separately and layer, or use a pastry bag and create a design.

DYSPHAGIA DIETS

When a **dysphagia diet** is necessary, this indicates there is a problem transferring the food from the mouth to the stomach or a problem swallowing. A swallowing evaluation is performed, and recommendations for food consistency are given by the speech–language pathologists base on the client's abilities. Foods may need to be thick or thin, smooth or textured, or light or heavy in consistency. You will be given specific guidelines for each client and for each type of food. No two clients will be the same. **Commercial thickeners** are sometimes used. Thin liquids tend to cause problems for clients.

- Find out how clients liked their food prepared before they had a problem with swallowing.
- Do not leave clients alone while they are eating.
- Be sure the food temperature is appropriate. Be sure the spices are appropriate. These clients cannot spit out a food that is too hot or too spicy.
- Be sure to notice any change in the client's ability to swallow.
- Be sure the client is sitting upright for meals.
- Feed slowly. *Do not* force clients to eat if they do not want to.

LOW-LACTOSE OR LACTOSE-FREE DIET

Lactose is a sugar found in dairy products. Many people are unable to digest lactose because they do not have the enzyme necessary to digest it. This problem usually runs in families, although all family members may not have it. This condition may be permanent or temporary. Lactose intolerance is considered a food allergy and should always be considered when preparing food.

Some people are able to tolerate small amounts of milk products. Others cannot tolerate any. When they eat anything that contains it, they suffer cramping, bloating, or diarrhea. People who suffer from this problem either eliminate all lactose from the diet and from food preparation or take medication prior to eating to aid in the digestion.

- Read labels to be sure that lactose is not in the food product.
- Identify the food products that can be used as substitutes for milk, such as rice milk or soy milk.
- When eating at restaurants or friends' homes, *ask* how the food is prepared.
- Do not encourage anyone to eat small amounts of lactose-containing food "to see if they still are allergic."

YOUR ROLE AS A HOMEMAKER/HOME HEALTH AIDE

As you help the client and family adjust to dietary modifications, the challenge will be to incorporate the modifications while still having the food be appetizing and satisfying to the client. Your encouragement and positive attitude will help the client accept the changes. Do not comment that the food does not appeal to you. Be aware of your facial expressions and body language as you serve the food or feed the client. Present the food as you would present any other meal in a cheerful, calm, and quiet environment. Do not change the consistency of the food without discussing the change with your supervisor. Even if the client appears to be able to swallow or tolerate different food, the prescribed diet can only be changed by the health care professional who manages the total care of the client.

POINTS TO REMEMBER

➢ Fiber is a natural part of a balanced diet, but the amount can be changed to meet a dietary need as calculated by a health professional.

➢ Monitoring the effects of dietary fiber, especially on the medication usually taken, is important and should be noted daily.

➢ Food intolerance should be taken seriously. Support clients as changes in their diet are made so as to meet their nutritional needs and allow them to view food as a positive part of their life.

➢ Diet modifications can be necessary for short or prolonged periods of time. Providing variety to your client is a challenge. Discuss this with your supervisor frequently.

CHAPTER 12

Food and Drug Interactions

Introduction

In this chapter, you will become familiar with the important role medications play in the total client's health. You will also become familiar with the way in which some foods could possibility interact with some medications and your role in being alert to these interactions. The timing of meals and medications is often a challenge and this chapter will present some suggestions for meeting this daily challenge in total client care.

People who take medication do so because they have a specific bodily need. These medications are prescribed by a health care professional for a specific reason. These professionals are licensed by the state to perform their duties. A person's unique reaction to medication depends on the general health of the individual, the medication, and the ability of the body to metabolize the medication and then process and dispose of the drug through the kidneys, liver, lungs, and skin. Often, the food we eat, however, does not cause a positive reaction when mixed with the medication in our bodies. The effect of a specific food and a specific medication can vary from person to person. Some people may be affected positively, some not at all, and some may have a negative reaction. When this occurs, the body may experience unpleasant and unexpected symptoms. The interactions of food and medication with alcohol and smoking is also a consideration. The interaction of food and medication pertains to *all* medications and drugs including over-the-counter drugs, herbal supplements, and vitamins and minerals. Prescription drugs are prescribed by a physician and cannot be bought without a prescription. Over-the-counter drugs can be bought without a prescription.

How Food and Drug Interactions Occur

Most food and drug interactions are the result of the interaction of oral medication and food. Oral drugs are swallowed and enter the stomach, where digestion is started. The partially digested substance passes to the small intestines, where the majority of absorption takes place. Further breakdown occurs as the remaining substances pass through the liver. The remaining undigested substances pass to the large intestines and are eliminated in the feces or to the kidneys and are eliminated through the urine.

- Food affects the absorption and emptying rate in the stomach.
- The stomach acid, although needed for digestion, may either break down the drug too quickly, speeding up absorption, or destroy the drug so that it is not useful to the body.
- Fatty foods may encourage the drug to remain in the stomach a long time and either delay absorption or promote the drug to be broken down to an unusable substance.
- Too much fiber may cause the drug to bind with it and alter absorption.

Drug Interactions

- Food can alter a drug's ability to work on the appropriate body system.
- Food can cause the drug to affect another body system.
- Food can cause the drug to work on the body system and cause a negative side effect.
- Food can cause toxic substances to form in the body.
- People most susceptible to food and drug interactions are the very young, the elderly, and debilitated people.

Drugs and the Elderly

Elderly clients react to medication differently than do younger clients. Often, elderly clients have several diseases and disabilities and take several medications. The interaction of all these medications and herbal supplements may produce unexpected side effects. Clients often save unused medication and take it when they think they need it.

Elderly clients face other situations that foster problems with medications:

- A client may forget having taken medications and repeat them or omit them altogether.
- A client may save medications that become outdated and then start taking them again.
- A client often has several physicians, each of whom may not be aware of all the medications that have been prescribed by other physicians.
- A client may stop taking medication for financial reasons.
- When your client visits a physician, encourage him to take all his medications with him.

BALANCING DRUG ADMINISTRATION WITH MEALS

Establishing a workable schedule of medication administration is an important activity you and your client will do together. Remember, if the schedule is easy to understand and adhere to, the client will maintain the schedule. If the schedule is not easy, the client will not keep to it. The main consideration is: Can the client maintain the schedule when you are not in the house? Assist your client with maintaining a safe medication schedule. Help your client maintain a foolproof, organized method of taking his medications. This method should be established by your supervisor with input from you and the client. Be sure all your client's medications and herbal supplements are prescribed for him. Borrowing medications can be dangerous! Report all side effects, no matter how slight, to your supervisor. If you and your client cannot establish a schedule, consult your supervisor, the pharmacist, or the physician.

When establishing a schedule, take the following into consideration by asking:

- What is the best time to take each medication?
- Are there any food and drug interactions, which should be considered?
- What supplements is the client taking such as vitamins, herbs, antacids, laxatives, and other medication? How will they all interact?

Discuss the schedule with the client, the family, and your supervisor.

THE FIVE RIGHTS OF MEDICATION ADMINISTRATION

To perform your duties well, you must know the Five Rights of Medication.

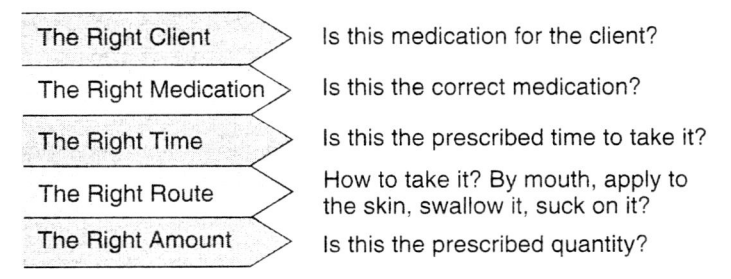

The Right Client	Is this medication for the client?
The Right Medication	Is this the correct medication?
The Right Time	Is this the prescribed time to take it?
The Right Route	How to take it? By mouth, apply to the skin, swallow it, suck on it?
The Right Amount	Is this the prescribed quantity?

FIGURE 12.1 The Five Rights of Medication must be observed every time a client takes medication.

MEDICATION LABELS

All medications have labels, which state clearly when a medication is to be taken and by whom. *It is not wise to take medication that is not specifically prescribed for the person taking it.* Usually, the medication bottles also have labels that indicate how the drug is to be taken: on a full stomach, before meals, after meals. Other considerations and possible side effects, such as drowsiness, are indicated. There are also indications of possible drug and food interactions and cautions to take into consideration. When a drugstore dispenses a prescription medication, the customer is usually given a sheet of paper with all this information on it. This should be kept in a safe, convenient place for further reference. When an over-the-counter drug is taken, this information can be found on the package. When herbal supplements are taken, the client may have to ask the pharmacist to identify any special considerations he or she will have to keep in mind while taking the substance.

MEDICATION STORAGE

- Clients save medication, but some of it changes its chemical makeup as it stands. Old medication should be disposed of with the client's permission.
- Many medications have similar names and look alike. Store these separately.
- Do not assist a client with a medication from an unlabeled container.
- Do not change the place your client stores his medication without his permission.
- Keep medication out of reach of children and confused, forgetful clients.

- Keep medication away from extreme heat, cold, or light.
- Encourage clients to throw out old, outdated medications and to return medications that are not theirs. Dispose of medication by flushing it down a toilet or pouring it down a drain.
- Help your clients get their medications packaged in containers that are easy for them to open and close. Often, clients will not take their medication because they cannot open the bottle. Be sure the medication is stored in a safe and easily used container.

Herbal Supplements

Many people do not consider herbal supplements medications. They are not considered medications, but they are substances that are digested by the body and cause some bodily change. It has been shown that many supplements can interact with prescribed medications and cause unexpected side effects. Some herbal supplements have information printed on the label and some do not. Some health care professionals ask about other medications being taken. Sometimes, clients will tell their physician when they are taking an herbal supplement, and sometimes they will not. The interactions of the supplements and the prescription and/or over-the-counter drugs is often not monitored by anyone because no one person knows about all of them.

General Guidelines of Common Food and Drug Interactions

Each drug affects each person differently. However, there are some broad guidelines, which should be taken into consideration when a specific drug is taken. There may be no need to be concerned with one client while another client will benefit from your questions and your alerting the family to the possibility of an interaction with food.

Drugs (Sampling—Not All Medications Included)

Antacids

- Continued use could alter calcium and phosphate levels in the blood.
- Large amounts could contribute to calcium loss and decreased bone integrity.
- Orange juice can alter **absorption.**
- Some are aluminum based and other magnesium based. Discuss the usefulness of taking one or the other.

Antibiotics

- Some are taken on an empty stomach; some are taken with food.
- Avoid wine, juice, soda, and dairy products when taking the medication
- Include yogurt during snack or meal times if possible.

Anticonvulsants

- Interferes with Vitamin D, calcium, vitamin B, and folic acid uptake by the body.
- The body's metabolism of the drug may alter over time.
- Avoid puddings.

Antidepressants

- May affect other drug absorption or effectiveness.
- Monoamine oxidase (MAO) inhibitors require the removal of all foods rich in tyramine, such as aged cheese, **miso** soup or soup base, yeast, pickled fish, avocado, pepperoni, salami, soy sauce, liver, chocolate, and caffeine.
- Grapefruit juice can alter absorption.

Antihistamines

- May affect appetite.
- May cause dry mouth or eyes.

Antihypertensives

- Some are taken with food, some without.
- Clients should discuss the use of ibuprofen with physician prior to taking it.

Asthma Medication

- Decrease charbroiled foods as they do not interact well with the medication.
- Avoid red peppers.

Aspirin

- Should be taken with food to decrease stomach irritation.
- Coated aspirin decreases stomach irritation.

- Clients taking aspirin over long periods of time may require vitamin C and/or iron supplements.
- Interaction with blood thinning drugs should be discussed.

Birth Control and Hormone Replacement

- May require Vitamin B_6 and folic acid supplement.

Blood-Thinning Drugs

- Foods rich in vitamin K and vitamin E such as broccoli, brussels sprouts, kale, asparagus, eggs and egg whites, lentils should be limited or avoided.
- Use of aspirin and aspirin-related drugs should be discussed with physician prior to taking them.

Chemotherapeutic Agents

- Cause appetite changes.
- Entire nutritional intake must be continually reviewed and altered to meet the body's needs.

Cholesterol-Lowering Drugs

- May alter absorption of fat-soluble vitamins requiring supplements.
- Should be taken with at least a large full glass of water.
- Some should be taken with food; some should be taken at night; others may be taken anytime.

Heart-Related Drugs

- May alter potassium and calcium balance in body.
- Highly alkaline foods such as milk, fruit, and vegetables should be reviewed by nutritionist.

Food (Partial Sample)

Bran and Oatmeal

- Alters digestion and absorption rate of all medication.

Milk

- Can make certain antibiotics, laxatives, and other medications useless.

Herbs (A Small Sampling of the Most Commonly Used)

Licorice (Used to Treat Colds and Respiratory Infections)

- This is found in some medication, candy, cough syrup, and herbal supplements. It can alter the absorption rate of all medications, causing unexpected side effects.
- Large amounts can also act as a laxative.
- Negative effects noted in those taking diabetes medications as it will interfere with the regulation of blood sugar levels.
- Negative effects noted in those taking heart medications as it will deplete the body of potassium.
- Can reduce the effect of thyroid medication.
- Interferes with many other organs such as kidney and liver.

Ginseng (Used to Increase Stamina and Boost Energy)

- May thin blood; therefore, do not take with heart, blood pressure, or diabetes medications.
- Do not take if taking any MAO inhibitors as it can cause mania.
- Increased irritability if mixed with caffeine.

Echinacea

This herb is used as an antibacterial and antiviral agent. It is used to treat colds and flu, claiming to boost the immune system.

- Do not take if on antifungal medications. This could injure the liver.
- Avoid if taking immune-suppressing drugs since the herb and drug perform opposite functions.
- Avoid if autoimmune, tuberculosis, multiple sclerosis, or acquired immune deficiency syndrome (AIDS) disease is present.

DRUGS AND ALCOHOL

Alcohol can affect drugs and the way they are absorbed and processed in the body. As a rule, alcohol and drugs of any kind should not be mixed. If you observe your client mixing these substances, report this to your supervisor immediately.

YOUR ROLE AS A HOMEMAKER/HOME HEALTH AIDE

Although you are not licensed to administer medication, you will be asked to assist your client, assist with scheduling, and be responsible for carefully observing your client after the medication has been taken.

Careful observation of your client is essential. You should also know the side effects of the medication, how to store the medication, and how it reacts with food. If you observe any side effects after your client has taken the medication, report them immediately to your supervisor. However, any change in behavior associated with the taking of medication should be noted.

Report to your supervisor immediately:

- If your client is not taking the medication exactly as it has been prescribed
- If your client is taking medication (prescription or over-the-counter) of which your supervisor is not aware
- If your client does not know why he is taking his drugs
- If his orientation, concentration, memory, or mood changes soon after he takes his medication
- If your client is confusing his medications

Different drugs can affect different people in a variety of ways. It is important for you to note and report any of the following reactions:

- Change in appetite (either increase or decrease)
- Stomach upset/nausea/vomiting
- Diarrhea
- Constipation
- Bloody stools or blood in the urine
- Dry mouth, aftertaste, or change in ability to taste food
- Change in body odor
- Change in salivation
- Change in skin, dry eyes, or bruising
- Change in vision
- Change in mental status, speech, or concentration

Be sure to report objectively, including:

- The time of your observation
- The relationship to the medication (before or after taking it)
- The duration of the symptoms
- What relieved it

- What you did
- What the client did
- Any subjective comments

> **POINTS TO REMEMBER**
>
> ➤ Food and drugs can interact positively or negatively in the body.
> ➤ Herbs should never be taken unless the physician prescribing the medications is aware of potential risks associated with the herbs and medications.
> ➤ Medication should be taken by the person for whom it is prescribed and exactly as it has been prescribed.
> ➤ Your role is to assist the client as he takes the medication and to carefully observe the effect it has on him. Report anything that is negative or unusual immediately!

CHAPTER 13

Feeding Difficulties and Alternatives

Introduction

In this chapter, you will find suggestions to meet everyday problems people face while eating. These problems can be present with all clients and with all types of diets. You will become familiar with how to observe changes. When you discuss them with your supervisor, both of you can agree to changes in the client's dietary regime. It is always wise to check with your supervisor before you institute changes no matter how small or insignificant you think they are.

Difficulties associated with nutrition, eating, and digestion are varied. Problems can occur because of physical reasons, medication, chemotherapy, or a combination of any of these. The results however, are usually the same: some disruption in the eating experience and some negative impact on total nutrition. Often, these disruptions can be addressed through a change in eating, timing of meals, timing of regular medication, or the type of food. Sometimes, however, additional medication may be needed to address the gastrointestinal disturbance and its results.

LOSS OF APPETITE

Changes in appetite are usual. Everyone does not have the same level of hunger or want the same type of food each day or even throughout the same day. However, when there is a significant change in appetite, this change must be noticed and addressed. Report changes as soon as they occur. These changes can be due to:

- Medication
- Emotional stress
- Physical stress
- Mental stress
- Pain
- Fatigue
- Poor-fitting dentures
- Difficulty breathing
- Difficulty swallowing
- Change in diet
- Allergies
- Eating disorder
- Chemotherapy
- Radiation therapy

It is helpful to try and identify the reason or reasons causing the appetite loss so that corrective action can be taken. Sometimes, however, it is difficult to identify one cause; therefore, all remedies must be tried.

BLOATING/EDEMA

Edema is caused by an imbalance between the fluid in the tissues and the fluid in the bloodstream. The bloating feeling can be limited to one part of the body such as the feet or hands, or it may be all over the body. It can affect the way a person breathes, walks, and sleeps. The edema may be due to a change in the function of one or more internal organs, protein imbalance, medication, or a change in a chronic disease.

This condition should be reported immediately to your supervisor. When you report it, make note of the following information, which will be helpful in determining the reason for the edema and possible actions that should be taken to remedy it:

- Where the edema is located
- The extent of the edema
- What is affected
- How long the condition has existed
- If it has occurred before, what relieved it

It is important to report this condition immediately. Do not assist the client with any change in medication or restrict fluids unless you are told to do so. Make the client comfortable while waiting.

Gas

Gas (flatus) is a normal by-product of digestion. Different people may find different foods to be gas producing. Most people know which foods case them discomfort. Respect this and take this into consideration when planning and cooking meals. Gas is not a problem unless the client is uncomfortable or cannot expel the gas. Then the condition should be reported immediately. A change in position or walking around may help relieve the condition.

Often, people who are prone to gas formation may find it helpful to limit gas producing foods such as:

Apples	Cabbage and related vegetables
Broccoli	Cauliflower
Carbonated drinks	Cucumbers
Corn	High-fiber foods
Milk and milk products	Turnips
Onions	
Bananas	

Sore Mouth or Throat

A sore mouth, gums, or throat may be due to an identified physical condition or medication that is being taken. It could also be caused by ill-fitting teeth. Once the cause is identified by the health care practitioner, medication often can be given to decrease the irritation. It is important to monitor this condition and not make light of it because it affects the client's nutritional and fluid intake. If you have concern, it is always wise to write down all food and fluid actually eaten so the client's nutritional intake can be accurately reviewed by your supervisor.

Certain foods, such as citrus juices and spicy foods, can irritate a sore mouth or throat. Soft foods may make it easier to chew and shallow. Sometimes liquids are taken for a day or two until the soreness subsides. Listen to the client and make of note of which foods irritate the condition and which do not. Listed below are suggestions to get you started. Add to this list as you discover other foods to include and avoid during times of sore mouth or throat (Table 13.1).

- Cold foods are usually more soothing than hot ones
- Cook foods until they are very soft and tender—almost mushy.
- Decrease the salt and spices used.

Table 13.1 Soft Foods to Include and Avoid with Sore Mouth or Throat

Foods to Include	Foods to Avoid
Cooked cereals like oatmeal	Orange juice
Cottage cheese	Grapefruit juice
Custards	Tangerines
Macaroni and cheese	Lemon juice
Mashed potatoes	Spicy foods
Milkshakes	Salty foods
Puddings	Raw vegetables
Scrambled eggs	Toast

NAUSEA/VOMITING

Nausea, either continual or occasional can be very upsetting and seriously impact the total nutritional intake and fluid balance of your client. Nausea can be related to medications, physical condition, chemotherapy, or radiation therapy. Some clients suffer nausea/vomiting often. The plan of care will have instructions on how to care for the client during these times.

Some foods can ease the uncomfortable feeling associated with nausea. The reaction to food is very individual. Your clients will tell you which foods make them sick. Often, a change in the timing of meals can also ease the nausea.

- Serve small meals.
- Try foods that are dry and crisp, such as crackers.
- Avoid fatty, greasy, and fried foods.
- Avoid smells that irritate the client.
- Explore a change in medication schedule.

Often, **vomiting** may follow nausea. Sometimes if nausea is controlled, vomiting can be avoided. If vomiting occurs, make the client comfortable and safe. Do not offer fluid or solid food until the vomiting is under control. Once the vomiting is under control, try small amounts of clear liquid such as ginger ale, chicken broth, or gelatin. Once clear liquids are tolerated, add some full-liquid diet foods such as cream soup, ice cream, or juice. The diet can be further advanced to soft foods such as plain chicken, macaroni and cheese, mashed potatoes, or cooked vegetables as the client feels better. The goal is to gradually add foods until back to "normal" eating habits. If altering food does not seem to help, relaxation exercises or even medication may help and be necessary.

It is important to report to your supervisor when a client has nausea and vomiting, especially if this is unusual so that an assessment can be made and a change in the care plan completed. It is important to manage nausea and vomiting when it first occurs so that **dehydration** can be avoided.

Constipation

Constipation is the inability of a person to expel fecal material. The cause may be a physical condition, diet, medication, or emotional state. However, the result is the same. Each person has different personal routine for evacuation of his bowels. Some people move their bowels daily, some every other day; some in the evening and some in the morning. It is important to know your client's usual routine and respect it. When constipation disrupts the usual routine, it should be reported and addressed. Severe constipation can result in abdominal discomfort and/or pain. It can also affect appetite, fluid balance, and medication absorption. Do not change medication or give over-the-counter laxatives. If, after consultation with your supervisor and health care professional, this is decided on, you and your client will make the necessary changes.

Food suggestions to prevent and decrease constipation include:

- Drink plenty of liquids—at least eight 8-ounce glasses every day. This will keeps stools soft. Fluid is also needed when fiber is increased in the diet.
- Eat fiber-rich foods, such as whole-grain products, fresh fruits and vegetables, and dried beans and peas. Eat the skin on fruits and potatoes. Add unprocessed wheat bran to foods like cereals, casseroles, and yogurt.
- Drink something hot about one half hour before your usual time for a bowel movement. This stimulates the bowel.
- Exercise every day, such as walking.

If these suggestions do not seem to help medication may be necessary to ease constipation.

Diarrhea

Diarrhea can be caused by infection, food sensitivity, medication, chemotherapy, radiation therapy, and even emotional upset. During diarrhea, food passes through the intestines rapidly before the body absorbs enough vitamins, minerals, and water. Prolonged diarrhea can result in dehydration, fluid imbalance, decreased appetite, change in physical activity, and abdominal pain. Report this condition to your supervisor. Be sure to report how long it has been going on, the frequency of the bowel movements, when it started, and if the cause is known. Do not assist the client in taking any medication to stop the diarrhea without speaking to your supervisor!

Signs and Symptoms of Dehydration

- Change in mental state: confusion, restlessness, excessive sleep
- Decreased urine output
- Fever
- Dry mouth and mucous membranes
- Dry, wrinkled skin that does not return to its position when lightly pinched

Food suggestions to decrease diarrhea include:

- Drink plenty of liquids in small amounts throughout the day. Drinking fluids will help replace what is lost.
- Eat plenty of foods and liquids rich in sodium and potassium. These minerals are essential and often lost through diarrhea. Foods high in sodium include broth and bouillon. Foods high in potassium that do not cause diarrhea include bananas, apricot and peach nectar, and mashed or boiled potatoes.
- Eat more low-fiber foods such as yogurt, cottage cheese, rice, noodles, ripe bananas, white bread, skinned chicken or turkey, lean beef, and fish. All food should be baked, broiled, or boiled.
- Avoid greasy, fatty, or fried foods of any kind.
- Avoid raw vegetables and fruits.
- Eliminate strong spices like curry and hot pepper.
- Limit foods and beverages that contain caffeine like coffee, strong tea, some sodas and chocolate.
- If a client is lactose intolerant be sure milk and milk products are not consumed.

ENTERAL NUTRITION

Clients who have a functioning gastrointestinal tract but cannot be adequately nourished by oral intake may need some other form of nutritional support. These clients will have **enteral** or tube feedings, which are put directly into the digestive tract through a tube. Tubes are used only for food and medication. The type of formula selected is based on the individual client's needs, tolerance, and condition. Many types of formulas are commercially available for use.

The type of tube feeding and the frequency and amount of the feeding will be determined by a nutritionist in consultation with a physician.

This is considered a prescription just as any medication is. Do not change it. If you have any concern about the tube feeding or you or the family have questions, ask the company that is responsible for bringing the product as well as your supervisor.

Most formulas are fortified with vitamins and minerals. Some are specialty formulas based on diseases, others are more concentrated and provide additional calories or proteins. Some are low in fiber and some are fiber enriched.

The client's condition and the length of time the tube feeding will be needed will often dictate the site selected for feeding tube. **Nasogastric** is often selected for short-term use. For longer use, a **gastrostomy** tube may be placed surgically into the stomach. When the stomach must be bypassed due to intractable vomiting, gastroesophageal reflux, or problems with gastric emptying, a surgically implanted **jejunostomy** tube may be used. Feeding may be continuous or intermittent. Continuous feedings permit a larger daily volume and less likelihood of diarrhea. These are usually tolerated best. Intermittent feeding will allow greater client mobility. Most formulas are administered by specially designed pumps, but gravity drip may also be used. Rate of administration will be determined by the prescription to meet the client needs.

You and the family will be instructed how to prepare the feeding, how to give the feeding, how to observe the client, and how to care for the equipment and the tube feeding. If you have questions, ask! Be sure you know the emergency telephone number of the company that prepares the feeding solution.

TOTAL PARENTERAL NUTRITION

When feeding by an enteral route is not possible, **total parenteral nutrition (TPN)** may be used. TPN is prepared in pharmacies under careful guidelines and with a physician prescription. The tube that is used for this feeding is not used for any other purpose. Some of the bottles or bags of TPN must be keep refrigerated until ready to hang. Feeding may be continuous or intermittent. Sometimes this is for a long period of time or could be short, usually not less than 5 days. If the gut is working, enteral nutrition is the preferred route of feeding. Your responsibility will be carefully discussed with you. You will be instructed in the care of the tube, the pump and the feeding. If you do not understand or have questions, ask!

YOUR ROLE AS A HOMEMAKER/HOME HEALTH AIDE

As you work with your clients and get to know them, you will observe their reaction to food. Your observations are important and should be shared regularly with your supervisor. Reactions to food are not always the same, so do not be surprised if your client suddenly develops one of the problems discussed in this chapter. By reporting any problems you notice or the client relates, you and your supervisor will be able to change the plan of care. Sometimes, a small change, such as the timing of a meal or the temperature of the food, will greatly increase the client's comfort. Be sure to report any problems you hear about that occur when you are not in the house.

POINTS TO REMEMBER

- Note and report all gastric disturbances in detail. Identifying the cause of them will help determine the best method of dealing with them.
- Changing a client's diet and/or feeding habits may often relieve gastric disturbances. These changes may have to be temporary or may have to continue for some length of time.
- Discuss changes with your client and your supervisor. Changes should be individualized for each client.
- Clients often must take medication to relieve gastric distress. Do not help clients take any medication, including over-the-counter medication, unless it has been prescribed specifically for them and you have been instructed to do so.

CHAPTER 14
Recipes for Soup

Introduction

Soup is a most versatile food. It may be used as the first course for a meal. It may be used as the main course of a meal, or it may even be used as a snack. Soup is easy to make, freezes well, and can be changed to meet the taste requirements and physical abilities of the client. Soup provides an easy way to obtain nutrition and is often one of the first foods offered to clients as they progress in their rehabilitation. Soups can be thick or thin, clear or creamed. Making soup is a very individual activity. You are encouraged to use these recipes as guides and to change the recipes to reflect the preferences of the client and of your experiences in relation to your client's preferences. You may also have to change the recipes to reflect the ingredients available due to time of the year. If your client likes the changes you make, note the changes in the book.

- When cooking soups, it is advisable to check the pot often to be sure that you have enough liquid in the pot. You may have to add some during the cooking process.
- Be careful when cooking and do not let the soups boil over.
- All soups should be stored in the refrigerator or the freezer.
- To reheat soup, bring the desired amount to a boil and boil for at least 2 minutes.

Recipes included in this chapter:

- Bean Soup
- Chicken Broth

- Lentil Soup
- Minestrone
- Split Pea Soup
- Tomato Soup
- Turkey Vegetable Soup
- Vegetable Soup

BEAN SOUP

Pre-Prep: 8 hours—soak beans
Prep time: 20 minutes

Cook time: 90 minutes
6 servings

Ingredients

1½ cups dry beans (navy, black, or cannelloni) picked over and soaked overnight in cold water (*Hint*: Change soaking water several times to reduce gas)

8 cups cold water
1 cup chopped onion
1 cup chopped celery
1 cup potatoes, peeled and chopped

Instructions

1. Bring cold water to a boil.
2. Add drained beans, onions, celery, and potatoes. Cover and bring to a boil.
3. Boil slowly about 2½–3 hours until beans are soft.
4. Puree if desired.

Nutrient Content

Calories 88
Protein 5 gm
20% calories from Protein
Carbohydrates 17 gm
Fat .28 gm

3% calories from Fat
Cholesterol 0 mg
Sodium 260 mg
Dietary Fiber 5 gm

Adaptations for Physical Limitations

- Adjust the consistency to the swallowing ability of the client by blending/pureeing soup before serving, or add thickening agent.

Substitutions

- Use **chicken stock** instead of water.
- Add ½ cup of diced **tomatoes** during the last 20 minutes of cooking.
- Use canned, cooked beans instead of dry beans, but decrease the cooking time by at least half.
- Vary the types of beans used.
- Add fully cooked, sliced **sausage** during the last 30 minutes of cooking.

Cultural Changes/Adaptations

- Add a small **ham** hock at time of cooking and remove before serving. Reserve the meat for another use or serve with soup.

CHICKEN BROTH

Prep time: 30 minutes
Cook time: 150 minutes

6 servings

Ingredients

- 1 chicken cleaned, quartered or whole
- 1 cup sliced onion
- 2 cups peeled carrots, cut into bite-size pieces
- 1 cup celery, cut into bite-size pieces
- 1 cup peeled parsnip, cut into bite-size pieces
- 6–8 cups cold water
- 2 tablespoons chopped dill
- 1 parsley root with parsley attached (optional)

Note: Chicken soup has many cultural variations. It is wise to discuss with the client and the family their personalization of the basic recipes.

Instructions

1. Put water in a large pot. Leave room for the chicken and vegetables. Bring to a boil.
2. Put the chicken, vegetables, and seasoning into the pot. Cover and bring to a boil.
3. Boil for about 1–1½ hours or until the chicken is soft. It may fall off the bone.
4. Remove the chicken into a bowl, taking care to save the soup as it drips out of the chicken.
5. You may also remove the vegetables.
6. a. The soup may be frozen at this point. The fat will rise to the top and can be scraped off before it is eaten.
   b. The soup may be eaten with or without the vegetable and pieces of chicken.
   c. The soup may be put into the refrigerator so the fat rises to the top and can be scraped off.
7. The chicken can be served with the soup, used later, made into chicken salad, or used in another dish.
8. The vegetables can be served with the soup, pureed and served separately, or pureed and put into the soup.

Nutrient Content

Calories 139
Protein 14 gm
40% calories from Protein
Carbohydrates 11 gm
Fat 4 gm

29% calories from Fat
Cholesterol 42 mg
Sodium 78 mg
Dietary Fiber 3 gm

Adaptations for Physical Limitations

- Adjust the consistency to the swallowing ability of the client by pureeing before serving or adding thickening agent as needed.

Substitutions

- Any *vegetables* can be cooked in the **broth** or added later.
- Serve with cooked **noodles,** cooked *rice,* or small ***macaroni.***

Cultural Changes/Adaptations

- Rapidly add a beaten *egg* to the rapidly boiling broth. Allow to cook for 45 seconds. Add 2 tablespoons *grated cheese.*
- Rapidly add 1 large beaten *egg* with 2 tablespoons lemon juice. Allow to cook 45 seconds.
- Cook 3–5 leaves of escarole in the broth until wilted. Add 2 tablespoons ***grated cheese.***
- Add diced fresh ginger after cooking.
- Add lemon during the last 30 minutes of cooking; remove before serving.

LENTIL SOUP

Prep time: 35 minutes
Cook time: 150 minutes

6 servings

Ingredients

1 tablespoon vegetable oil
8 cups water
1 ham bone (optional) or ½ pound ham, cooked
1 cup chopped celery
1 cup chopped onion

1 cup carrots, peeled and chopped
1 bay leaf
2 tablespoons chopped parsley
1 teaspoon chopped thyme
1½ cups lentils, picked over and washed

Instructions

1. In a medium-size pot, heat the oil and sauté the onion, celery, and carrots until wilted, about 8–10 minutes.
2. Add the water, bay leaves, parsley, thyme, and lentils. If the ham bone is used, add this too.
3. Add enough water to cover the contents.
4. Cover and simmer for 1-1½ hours. Check the pot often. Stir the contents and add water as necessary to keep the contents a soupy consistency. If too much liquid, continue to boil.
5. Remove the ham bone and bay leaves.
6. The soup can be eaten if this is the consistency desired. If not, puree the soup while it is still warm. Use a mixer or egg beater, or force the contents through a sieve or food mill.

Nutrient Content

Calories 269
Protein 23 gm
33% calories from Protein
Carbohydrates 33 gm
Fat 6 gm

19% calories from Fat
Cholesterol 22 mg
Sodium 566 mg
Dietary Fiber 16 gm

Adaptations for Physical Limitations

- Adjust the consistency to the swallowing ability of the client by pureeing before serving or adding thickening agent as needed.

Substitutions

- Add 2 cups chopped **tomatoes**.
- Substitute **chicken or beef stock** for water.
- Wash and cut up ½ bunch of greens, spinach, mustard greens, or kale. Cook in finished soup until tender.
- Add 1 large diced **potato** and ½ cup water 30 minutes before soup is finished.

Cultural Changes/Adaptations

- Omit the ham bone or **ham**.
- Any type of **sausage** can be added instead of or in addition to the **ham**.

MINESTRONE

Prep time: 30 minutes
Cook time: 90 minutes

8 servings

Ingredients

1 tablespoon olive or vegetable oil
1½ cups diced onion
1 cup diced celery
1 cup carrots, peeled and diced
2–4 leaves of green cabbage, shredded (optional)
4 cloves garlic, peeled and diced
10 cups water
1 bay leaf
1 teaspoon thyme
1 teaspoon basil
1 tablespoon parsley
1 14.5-ounce can tomatoes mashed into small size pieces
1 15.5-ounce can garbanzo beans, drained
1 15.5-ounce can pinto, white, or kidney beans, drained
¾ cup macaroni, orzo, shells, or small pasta

Instructions

1. Heat the oil in a soup pot. Add onions, celery, and carrots. Cook until limp, about 7 minutes
2. Add cabbage, garlic, water, bay leaf, thyme, basil, parsley, and tomatoes. Cook about 3 minutes.
3. Carefully add the water. Cover. Bring to a boil and simmer for 45 minutes.
4. Add the beans. Cook 20 minutes.
5. Add the pasta and cook until the pasta is soft, about 5–7 minutes.
6. Remove the bay leaf before serving.

Nutrient Content

Calories 81
Protein 3 gm
14% calories from Protein
Carbohydrates 14 gm
Fat 2 gm
22% calories from Fat
Cholesterol 0 mg
Sodium 106 mg
Dietary Fiber 3 gm

Adaptations for Physical Limitations

- Adjust the consistency to the swallowing ability of the client by pureeing before serving or adding thickening agent as needed.

Substitutions

- Use *chicken stock* instead of water.
- Vary the beans.
- Vary the greens, using spinach, dandelion greens, or collard greens.
- Add *sausage* or any leftover meat.
- Rice may be used in place of macaroni.
- Serve with a sprinkling of *grated cheese*.

SPLIT PEA SOUP

Prep time: 30 minutes
Cook time: 120 minutes

6 servings

Ingredients

2 tablespoons vegetable oil
1 cup chopped onion
½ cup chopped celery
¾ cup carrots, peeled and chopped into small pieces
10 cups low-sodium chicken broth
2 bay leaves

2 tablespoons parsley
¾ cup potatoes, peeled and cut into small pieces
1 cup green split peas (yellow split peas can be used with the green ones)
1 ham bone with meat on it (bone with about 3 ounces of meat, optional)

Instructions

1. In a medium-size pot, heat the oil and sauté the onion, celery, and carrots until wilted, about 8–10 minutes.
2. Add the chicken broth, bay leaves, parsley, potatoes, and split peas. If the ham bone is used, add this too.
3. If necessary, add just enough water to cover all the ingredients in the pot.
4. Cover and simmer for 2–2½ hours. Check the pot often. Stir the contents and add water as necessary to keep the contents a soupy consistency. If too much liquid, continue to boil. Cook until the peas are liquefied.
5. Remove the ham bone and bay leaves.
6. The soup can be eaten if this is the consistency desired. If not, puree the soup while it is still warm. Use a mixer or egg beater, or force the contents through a sieve or food mill.

Nutrient Content

Calories 275
Protein 18 gm
26% calories from Protein
Carbohydrates 31 gm
Fat 9 gm

30% calories from Fat
Cholesterol 19 mg
Sodium 420 mg
Dietary Fiber 10 gm

Adaptations for Physical Limitations

- Adjust the consistency to the swallowing ability of the client by pureeing before serving, adding more liquid, or adding thickening agent as needed.

Substitutions

- Use water, **vegetable juice,** or **regular chicken broth** instead of low-sodium chicken broth.
- Use 2–4 tablespoons chopped cooked **ham** instead of ham bone.

Cultural Changes/Adaptations

- Omit the **ham** bone and chopped cooked **ham** for kosher clients.

TOMATO SOUP

Prep time: 10 minutes
Cook time: 30 minutes

6 servings

Ingredients

1 tablespoon olive or vegetable oil
½ medium onion, finely chopped
1 28-ounce can tomatoes peeled
  and chopped

5–6 cups water

Instructions

1. Heat the oil in a soup pot. Cook the onions until limp, about 10–15 minutes.
2. Add the tomatoes and water. Cook covered at a slow boil. Cook 20–30 minutes.
3. Cool about 45 minutes.
4. Puree in a blender or force through a sieve or food mill.
5. Return to the pot and heat until warm.

Nutrient Content

Calories 64
Protein 2 gm
12% calories from Protein
Carbohydrates 10 gm
Fat 3 gm

33% calories from Fat
Cholesterol 0 mg
Sodium 181 mg
Dietary Fiber 3 gm

Adaptations for Physical Limitations

- Adjust the consistency to the swallowing ability of the client by adding more liquid or adding thickening agent as needed.

Substitutions

- Use **chicken stock** instead of water.
- Add ½ cup **milk** and heat.
- Add **croutons** before serving.
- Sprinkle with **grated cheese** prior to serving.
- May add 1 cup cooked **small pasta** or cooked **rice** when reheating.
- Add **sour cream** or **fat-free sour cream** at serving time.
- Add 1 tablespoon chopped basil at time of serving.
- Add 1 tablespoon chopped cilantro at time of serving.

TURKEY VEGETABLE SOUP

Prep time: 40 minutes
Cook time: 60 minutes

6 servings

Ingredients

- 1 roasted turkey carcass or part of one cooked without most of the meat or stuffing
- 10 cups cold water
- 3 carrots, peeled and chopped
- 1 cup onion, peeled and chopped
- ¾ cup chopped celery
- ½ cup parsnips, peeled and chopped
- 1 cup chopped zucchini
- 1½ cup potatoes, peeled and chopped
- ½ cup frozen green peas
- ½ cup frozen green beans
- 1 cup chopped canned tomatoes (optional)
- 1 bay leaf
- ½ tablespoon chopped parsley

Instructions

1. Put water in a large pot. Leave room for the turkey and vegetables. Bring to a boil.
2. Put the turkey and vegetables and all seasoning into the pot. Cover and bring to a boil.
3. Boil for about 1 hour or until the vegetables are soft and the majority of the meat has fallen off the turkey carcass.
4. Remove the turkey to a bowl, taking care to save the soup as it drips from the turkey. Remove the bay leaf.
5. You may remove the vegetables also.
6. a. The soup may be frozen at this point. The fat will rise to the top and can be scraped off before it is eaten.
   b. The soup may be eaten with or without the vegetables and pieces of turkey.
   c. The soup may be put into the refrigerator so the fat rises to the top and can be scraped off.
7. The turkey can be served with the soup. If there is enough meat, it can be used later, made into turkey salad or turkey pot pies.
8. The vegetables can be pureed and served with the soup or served separately.

Nutrient Content

Calories 110
Protein 5 gm
16% calories from Protein
Carbohydrates 21 gm
Fat 1 gm

11% calories from Fat
Cholesterol 6 mg
Sodium 112 mg
Dietary Fiber 5 gm

Adaptations for Physical Limitations

- Adjust the consistency to the swallowing ability of the client by pureeing the vegetables, adding more liquid, or adding thickening agent as needed.

Substitutions

- Use **vegetable stock** instead of water.
- Add small cooked **pasta, rice,** or **orzo**.
- Add **turnips, mushrooms,** or **hot peppers**.

VEGETABLE SOUP

Prep time: 30 minutes
Cook time: 90 minutes

8 servings

Ingredients

¼ cup diced onion
1 cup carrots, peeled and diced
¾ cup diced celery
1 cup potatoes, peeled and diced
4 cups frozen mixed vegetables
10 cups water

1 bay leaf
1 teaspoon thyme
1 tablespoon parsley
1 28-ounce can tomatoes mashed into bite-size pieces
Salt and pepper to taste

Instructions

1. Put water in a large pot. Leave room for the vegetables. Bring to a boil.
2. Add vegetables. Cover and return to a boil.
3. Boil about 60 minutes or until the vegetables are tender.
4. Remove the bay leaf.
5. Puree if desired.

Nutrient Content

Calories 131
Protein 6 gm
17% calories from Protein
Carbohydrates 29 gm
Fat 1 gm

6% calories from Fat
Cholesterol 0 mg
Sodium 227 mg
Dietary Fiber 8 gm

Adaptations for Physical Limitations

- Adjust the consistency to the swallowing ability of the client by pureeing the vegetables, adding more liquid, or adding thickening agent as needed.

Substitutions

- Use **chicken stock** or **beef stock** instead of water.
- Vary the beans.
- Serve with a sprinkling of **grated cheese.**
- Add **turnips, mushrooms, or hot peppers** during the cooking.
- Add leftover meat. Heat before serving.
- Add 2 cups cooked **rice or pasta.**
- Add **precooked sausage** after first 30 minutes of cooking. Cook well.

CHAPTER 15

Recipes for Entrées: Beef, Lamb, Pork, Poultry, Fish, and Meatless

Introduction for Beef

Beef is the most popular meat eaten in the United States. Within the past 10 years, in response to the health needs of Americans, beef has become much leaner and is now included in many more diets. Meat is inspected and graded according to government standards. The highest grade of meat is Prime. This has the highest fat content of all grades. It is also the most tender after cooking. The most common grade of meat is Choice. This is the usual grade sold in most supermarkets. Some meat is ungraded and must be chosen by looking at it. Some meats have labels such as "organic," "natural," or "free-range." It is important to know how each label is defined.

The tenderest cuts of meat are the rib, loin, and sirloin and can be broiled or pan broiled. The tougher cuts of meat—chuck, brisket, shank, and rump—must be moist cooked a long time as pot roasts or stews. It is important to become familiar with names given to cuts of meat in your area since some cuts of meat have different names in different areas of the country.

Changing the seasoning when cooking will greatly change the flavor of the finished dish. The following seasonings are particularly useful when cooking beef. Try them in small quantities in varying combinations:

Dry mustard	Marjoram
Thyme	Bay leaf (remove before eating)
Pepper	Parsley
Curry	Orange rind
Ginger	Garlic
Mushroom	Onion
Red pepper	Green pepper
Chilies	

Different people prefer meat cooked to varying degrees of doneness. Some people like rare meat, some like it pink, and some like it well done with no pink visible. Some people like fat left on their meat and some people remove all visible fat before cooking. When roasting any meat, to reduce the amount of fat eaten, roast the meat on a rack. Discuss this with your client, and take the family preference into consideration when preparing and planning meals. You may meet people who like to eat raw meat. Usually, this is not recommended as it may contain some bacteria that would ordinarily be killed during cooking. Discuss this preference with your supervisor.

Recipes included in this section of this chapter:

- Beef Stew (Quick)
- Chili
- Meatloaf
- Pepper Steak
- Pot Roast
- Sloppy Joes

BEEF STEW (QUICK)

Prep time: 15 minutes
Cook time: 60 minutes

6 servings

Ingredients

Vegetable oil spray
¾ pound (12 ounces) beef stew cubes
½ cup minced onion
½ cup minced celery
½ cup minced carrots
2 cups cooking liquid: beef broth, chicken broth, vegetable broth, or water

15 ounces canned tomatoes
1 package dry onion soup mix
2 cup sliced potatoes
1 cup green beans

Instructions

1. Heat a large pot, spray bottom with vegetable oil spray.
2. Brown the meat thoroughly on all sides (about 10 minutes). Remove the meat to a platter.
3. Brown the onions, celery and carrots (about 7 minutes).
4. Return the meat to the pan and add the liquid, tomatoes, and the onion soup mix. Cook covered for about 1–1½ hours. The meat should be tender when a fork can be inserted easily.
5. Add the potatoes and green beans and cook another 15–20 minutes.

Nutrient Content

Calories 220
Protein 14 gm
25% calories from Protein
Carbohydrates 18 gm
Fat 10.5 gm

43% calories from Fat
Cholesterol 38 mg
Sodium 1023 mg
Dietary Fiber 3 gm

Adaptations for Physical Limitations

- Adjust the consistency to the swallowing ability of the client by cutting the meat into small pieces or pureeing the food once it has completed the cooking process. Add liquid or a thickening agent if necessary.

Substitutions

- Add **vegetables** of choice.
- Use 2 tablespoons **vegetable oil** in place of vegetable oil spray.
- Add cayenne pepper to taste.
- Vary cooking liquid using **beef broth, vegetable broth.**
- Add **dried fruit** when the meat is about halfway done.
- Add garlic for flavor when cooking.
- Leave **tomatoes** out of the recipe.

CHILI

Prep time: 20 minutes
Cook time: 40 minutes

4 servings

Ingredients

- 1 cup cooked kidney beans
- 1 tablespoon vegetable oil
- 1 cup onion, chopped
- 1 clove minced garlic or $\frac{1}{2}$ teaspoon garlic powder
- 12 ounces ($\frac{3}{4}$ pound) lean ground beef
- 1 tablespoon oregano
- 3 tablespoons chili seasoning powder
- $\frac{1}{4}$ teaspoon black pepper
- $\frac{1}{4}$ teaspoon ground cumin
- $1\frac{1}{2}$ cups tomato sauce—no salt added
- $1\frac{1}{2}$ tablespoons cider vinegar

Instructions

1. Heat the kidney beans according to the package. Do not add salt.
2. Heat oil in deep pot or skillet over medium heat.
3. Add the onion and garlic, and sauté until soft.
4. Add the beef. Continue to stir with fork to break the meat up as it continues to brown.
5. Stir in seasoning, tomatoes, and vinegar.
6. Add the beans and mix well.
7. Reduce heat to low and cook covered for additional 30 minutes, stirring occasionally.

Nutrient Content

Calories 368
Protein 20 gm
22% calories from Protein
Carbohydrates 22 gm
Fat 21 gm

53% calories from Fat
Cholesterol 64 mg
Sodium 245 mg
Dietary Fiber 7 gm

Adaptations for Physical Limitations

- Adjust the consistency to the swallowing ability of the client by cutting the meat into small pieces or pureeing the food once it has completed the cooking process. Add liquid or a thickening agent if necessary.

Substitutions

- Any combination of ground meat can be used *(turkey, chicken, veal, pork)*.
- Excess fat can be drained from meat prior to adding seasonings and tomatoes.
- Any cooked *beans* can be used in place of or in addition to kidney beans.
- Serve with *grated cheese* on top.

MEATLOAF

Prep time: 20 minutes
Cook time: 60 minutes

4 servings

Ingredients

12 ounces (¾ pound) lean ground beef
¼ cup onion, chopped
¼ cup canned tomato sauce—low sodium
1 large egg, slightly beaten

½ cup plain bread crumbs
1 tablespoon dried parsley
½ teaspoon ground black pepper
Vegetable oil spray

Instructions

1. In a bowl, combine beef, onion, tomato sauce, egg, and bread crumbs.
2. Mix parsley and pepper together. Add to meat mixture.
3. Mix all ingredients well.
4. Spray an 8- or 9-inch loaf pan with vegetable oil spray.
5. Pack and press the mixture down in the loaf pan. Smooth out the top.
6. Bake in preheated 350° oven for 1 hour.
7. Remove meat from pan. Serve.

Nutrient Content

Calories 266
Protein 19 gm
29% calories from Protein
Carbohydrates 12 gm
Fat 15 gm

53% calories from Fat
Cholesterol 59 mg
Sodium 191 mg
Dietary Fiber .6 gm

Adaptations for Physical Limitations

- Adjust the consistency to the swallowing ability of the client by cutting the meat into small pieces or pureeing the food once it has completed the cooking process. Add liquid or a thickening agent if necessary.

Substitutions

- Any combination of ground meat can be used *(turkey, chicken, veal, pork).*
- **Ketchup** can be substituted for tomato sauce.

PEPPER STEAK

Prep time: 20 minutes
Cook time: 50 minutes

5 servings

Ingredients

1 pound round steak, skirt steak, or flank steak
Vegetable oil spray
1 cup minced onion
1 teaspoon minced garlic
1 cup green pepper, seeded and minced

1 $14\frac{1}{2}$-ounce can of beef broth
$1\frac{1}{2}$ tablespoons cornstarch
2 teaspoons soy sauce
$\frac{1}{4}$ cup water

Instructions

1. Slice the meat into very thin slices (sliced on the diagonal). (Put the meat in the freezer for 30 minutes before slicing to make this easier.)
2. In a large skillet, heat the oil. Brown the meat, garlic, and onions.
3. Add the green pepper and beef broth. Cook covered for 10 minutes.
4. Mix the cornstarch, soy sauce, and water in a small dish. Add this to the pot and until the liquid is thickened.
5. Adjust seasoning.

Nutrient Content

Calories 189
Protein 19 gm
40% calories from Protein
Carbohydrates 6 gm
Fat 10 gm

47% calories from Fat
Cholesterol 47 mg
Sodium 199 mg
Dietary Fiber 1 gm

Adaptations for Physical Limitations

- Adjust the consistency to the swallowing ability of the client by cutting the meat into small pieces or pureeing the food once it has completed the cooking process. Add liquid or a thickening agent if necessary.

Substitutions

- Add additional **vegetables** of choice.
- Use small **chicken or pork** cubes instead of beef. Adjust cooking time.
- 2 tablespoons **vegetable oil** may be used in place of vegetable oil spray.

POT ROAST

Prep time: 20 minutes
Cook time: 120 minutes

6 servings

Ingredients

2 tablespoons vegetable oil
2 pounds of meat: rump, chuck, or brisket
1½ cup minced onion
½ cup minced celery
½ cup minced carrots

2 cups beef broth
1 bay leaf
1 tablespoon dried dill
3 tablespoons ketchup
1 15-ounce can of tomatoes (optional)

Instructions

1. Remove all visible fat from the meat.
2. Heat the oil in a large pot, and brown the meat on all sides. Remove the meat to a platter. Brown the onions, celery, and carrots in the pan, about 7 minutes.
3. Return the meat to the pan.
4. Add the broth, ketchup, dill, and bay leaf carefully so the broth doesn't splatter.
5. Cook covered for about 1½ hours. The meat is tender when a fork can be inserted easily.
6. Add the tomatoes and cook another 10 minutes.
7. Remove bay leaf before serving.

Nutrient Content

Calories 323
Protein 23 gm
28% calories from Protein
Carbohydrates 6 gm
Fat 23 gm

65% calories from Fat
Cholesterol 76 mg
Sodium 342 mg
Dietary Fiber 1 gm

Adaptations for Physical Limitations

- Adjust the consistency to the swallowing ability of the client by cutting the meat into small pieces or pureeing the food once it has completed the cooking process. Add liquid or a thickening agent if necessary.

Substitutions

- In place of beef broth, any of the following may be used: **chicken broth, vegetable broth**, or **water**.
- Add **vegetables** of choice or peeled **potato** chunks when adding the tomatoes.
- Add cayenne pepper to taste.
- Add **dried fruit** when the meat is about halfway done.
- Add garlic when cooking.
- Use **vegetable oil spray** in place of liquid vegetable oil.

SLOPPY JOES

Prep time: 10 minutes
Cook time: 60 minutes

4 servings

Ingredients

1 pound lean ground beef
2 cups tomato sauce—no salt added
½ cup chopped onion

1 sloppy joe seasoning packet
4 hamburger buns

Instructions

1. Simmer beef for about 40 minutes. Chop and crumble meat with fork, stirring often as it browns.
2. Add tomato sauce, onions, and seasoning packet. Cook until the meat is completely cooked.
3. Serve open faced on hamburger bun.

Nutrient Content

Calories 403
Protein 25 gm
24% calories from Protein
Carbohydrates 37 gm
Fat 18 gm

40% calories from Fat
Cholesterol 69 mg
Sodium 1029 mg
Dietary Fiber 1 gm

Adaptations for Physical Limitations

- Adjust the consistency to the swallowing ability of the client by pureeing the food once it has completed the cooking process. Add liquid or a thickening agent if necessary.

Substitutions

- Eliminate *onions* if desired.
- Use crock pot for extended slow cooking.
- For milder flavor, use only ½ packet of *seasoning mix*.
- Serve with grated *cheddar cheese* on top.

Introduction for Lamb

Lamb is available in all parts of the United States. When buying lamb, it is important to identify if it is American lamb, New Zealand lamb, or Australian lamb. New Zealand and Australian lamb are usually smaller. American lamb is generally considered the most tender and is usually available fresh. Lamb is graded either prime, choice, or good. Most of what is available in the supermarkets is choice. Prime lamb is available from very exclusive butchers.

Lamb can be very fatty. All visible fat should be removed before cooking, as should the thin white membrane called the fell. By removing the fell and the fat, the seasoning can penetrate the meat and the drippings will be less fatty.

- Lamb is often eaten rare or medium, depending on the client preference.
- Mint jelly is often served with the roasted or broiled cuts of meat.

Recipes included in this section of this chapter:

- Braised Lamb Shanks
- Lamb Chops

BRAISED LAMB SHANKS

Prep time: 20 minutes
Cook time: 60 minutes

2 servings

Ingredients

2 lamb shanks, about 1 pound each
1 cup chopped onion
1 cup chopped carrot
$\frac{1}{2}$ cup chopped celery
1 teaspoon paprika
1 teaspoon garlic powder
$\frac{1}{2}$ teaspoon rosemary
6 ounces tomato juice
2 cups water
Vegetable oil spray

Instructions

1. Spray a heavy skillet or pot with vegetable oil and heat.
2. Place the lamb shanks in the pot and brown on all sides. If the lamb sticks, add a small amount of water as the meat browns.
3. Remove from the pot.
4. Add the onions, carrots, and celery, Cook until wilted.
5. Return the lamb to the pot with any juices.
6. Add the spices, tomato juice, and water.
7. Cover and cook about 1 hour or until the meat is tender.

Nutrient Content

Calories 322
Protein 42 gm
53% calories from Protein
Carbohydrates 19 gm
Fat 8 gm
23% calories from Fat
Cholesterol 133 mg
Sodium 425 mg
Dietary Fiber 4 gm

Adaptations for Physical Limitations

- Adjust the consistency to the swallowing ability of the client by cutting the meat into small pieces or pureeing the food once it has completed the cooking process. Add liquid or a thickening agent if necessary.

Substitutions

- Add additional *root vegetables* such as *parsnips* or *turnips*.
- Add red pepper for additional spice.
- Use *beef broth* or *vegetable broth* instead of water.
- Use *tomato sauce* instead of tomato juice.

LAMB CHOPS

Prep time: 10 minutes
Cook time: 15 minutes

2 servings

Ingredients

1 shoulder lamb chop per person or 2 to 3 rib or loin chops per person
½ cup water

Rosemary or thyme (optional)
Vegetable oil spray

Instructions

Broiling Method

1. Preheat broiler for 5 minutes.
2. Line the broiler pan with aluminum foil.
3. Place broiler rack and pan so it is about 5 inches from the heat source.
4. Place 2 tablespoons of water in the bottom of the pan to prevent the grease from spattering.
5. Season the lamb chops with rosemary, thyme, salt, and pepper if desired.
6. Place lamb chops on the broiler pan. Cook for about 5 minutes per side. This time may be more or less depending on the way the client likes the meat and the distance from the heat source.

Pan-Broiled Method

1. Heat a heavy skillet. You may wish to spray it with vegetable oil spray. Arrange the seasoned chops in a skillet.
2. Cook for about 4–5 minutes per side depending on how the client likes the meat.
3. Serve immediately.

Nutrient Content

Calories 112
Protein 17 gm
65% calories from Protein
Carbohydrates 0 gm
Fat 4 gm

35% calories from Fat
Cholesterol 54 mg
Sodium 56 mg
Dietary Fiber 0 gm

Adaptations for Physical Limitations

- Adjust the consistency to the swallowing ability of the client by cutting the meat into small pieces or pureeing the food once it has completed the cooking process. Add liquid or a thickening agent if necessary.

Substitutions

- Use various spices such as dill, chives, garlic, or hot pepper.
- Serve with mint *jelly.*

Introduction for Pork

In some parts of the country, pork is the most common meat. While some cultures do not eat pork at all, others eat it more than any other food. Pork used to be cooked a very long time and never eaten the slightest bit pink. This was so that all traces of disease would be removed. Today, with all meat being inspected and with new knowledge about diseases, pork, above the temperature of 137°, is disease free.

Recipes included in this section of this chapter:

- Pork Medallions
- Pork Stir-Fry

PORK MEDALLIONS

Prep time: 15 minutes
Cook time: 15 minutes

2 servings

Ingredients

8 ounces pork tenderloin
2 tablespoon olive oil

4 tablespoons flour
3 tablespoons lemon juice

Instructions

1. Cut the tenderloin into thin pieces about $\frac{1}{2}$-inch thick. If you freeze the meat for 30 minutes, it will be easier to cut.
2. Put the flour into a flat dish.
3. Heat the oil in a skillet.
4. Coat the pork with the flour and sauté in the oil until done.
5. Remove to a plate and keep covered.
6. Pour lemon juice into the pan. Remove all the drippings and pour over the pork.

Nutrient Content

Calories 339
Protein 25 gm
30% calories from Protein
Carbohydrates 14 gm
Fat 20 gm

54% calories from Fat
Cholesterol 75 mg
Sodium 59 mg
Dietary Fiber 0 gm

Adaptations for Physical Limitations

- Adjust the consistency to the swallowing ability of the client by cutting the meat into small pieces or pureeing the food once it has completed the cooking process. Add liquid or a thickening agent if necessary.

Substitutions

- Vary spices used on the meat.
- May use ***chicken, beef, or veal*** instead of pork or as a combination. Change the cooking time as needed.
- Marinate meat for 30 minutes in ***soy sauce, balsamic vinegar,*** or ***flavored vinegar.*** Discard the marinade.
- Use flavored vinegar instead of lemon juice.
- Vary oils to include peanut, sesame, or flavored oils.
- Add 2 tablespoons of ***peanuts, walnuts,*** or ***pine nuts*** at the end of the cooking.
- Add any combination of raw ***vegetables*** to cook after the meat.

PORK STIR-FRY

Prep time: 15 minutes
Cook time: 15 minutes

4 servings

Ingredients

8-ounce pork tenderloin
1 teaspoon vegetable oil
1 tablespoon soy sauce

1 teaspoon grated ginger
1 teaspoon garlic powder
½ cup snow pea pods

Instructions

1. Cut the tenderloin into thin pieces about ½-inch thick. If you freeze the meat for 30 minutes, it will be easier to cut.
2. Heat the oil in the skillet.
3. Cook the meat and remove to a plate. Keep warm.
4. Add the snow peas. When snow peas are cooked, return the meat to the pan and add the soy sauce, gingerroot, and garlic powder.
5. Heat all ingredients together until hot and serve.

Nutrient Content

Calories 235
Protein 25 gm
42% calories from Protein
Carbohydrates 4 gm
Fat 13 gm

51% calories from Fat
Cholesterol 75 mg
Sodium 716 mg
Dietary Fiber 1 gm

Adaptations for Physical Limitations

- Adjust the consistency to the swallowing ability of the client by cutting the meat into small pieces or pureeing the food once it has completed the cooking process. Add liquid or a thickening agent if necessary.

Substitutions

- Vary *oils* to include *peanut, sesame,* or flavored.
- Add *sesame seeds* at the end of cooking.
- Any combination of *raw vegetable* can be used.
- Any flavoring sauce such as hoisin, fish sauce, curry, garlic, or curry paste can be used at the end of cooking.
- Use low sodium *soy sauce* instead of regular soy sauce.

Introduction for Chicken

Chicken is a very versatile food. It is also comparatively inexpensive. You will find that chicken is a part of almost very diet. Your challenge is to assist your client in planning meals that have variety and taste.

Chickens are raised in a variety of ways. They are often labeled "free-range," "organic," or "natural." It is wise to find out what each processor means by these terms as they vary from brand to brand and area to area. Self-basting chickens and turkeys mean that the processor has inserted fat under the skin to flavor the meat.

Kosher chickens are slaughtered under the supervision of a rabbi and then prepared for selling. Halal chickens are slaughtered under the supervision of someone of the Islamic faith and then prepared for selling. If your client requests the purchase of one of these chickens, respect his or her wishes and do not substitute another for it.

When buying poultry:

- Check sell date. Never buy a package past the sell date. You may freeze chicken if necessary but never initially freeze a package past the sell date.
- Color is not an indication of the freshness of the chicken as color can be changed by changing the feed of the birds. If you open the package and it does not have a fresh smell, do not eat it! Either return it immediately or throw it out.
- Determine whether the chicken was been frozen before you bought it. Do not refreeze unless you cook it and then freeze it.

When storing poultry:

- Store poultry on the bottom shelf of the refrigerator so it cannot drip on anything else. Always store it in a dish that can be washed.
- Thaw in cold water or the refrigerator before cooking. Do not thaw poultry on the counter.
- Poultry can be defrosted in the microwave very carefully so as not to cook it.
- Always store poultry covered.

When cooking poultry:

- Cut poultry on an acrylic cutting board. Do not touch raw poultry and then touch something else. Wash all utensils after using them in hot, soapy water before using them for anything else!
- Usually, poultry should be defrosted before it is cooked; however, some prepared items go from the freezer to the oven. Read labels.
- Cook poultry until no blood is evident.

- Internal temperatures of a cooked chicken or turkey should be measured by an accurate thermometer:
  - White meat should be 160°.
  - Dark meat, thigh and leg 180°.
  - Juices should run clear when pricked with a fork.
- Stuffing whole birds and turkey breasts should be done right before the bird goes into the oven. Do not store a stuffed bird in the refrigerator.
  - Stuffing should be 160° before it is removed from the oven.
  - Pack the stuffing loosely into the cavity.
  - Remove the stuffing from the bird before carving.

Seasonings particularly useful when varying the taste of chicken dishes are:

Curry	Turmeric
Cumin	Cilantro
Tarragon	Thyme
Sage	Garlic
Ginger	Orange, lemon, or lime juice
Mushrooms	Onions
Tomatoes	

Recipes included in this section of this chapter:

- Boneless Chicken Breast Sautéed
- Chicken Cutlets Breaded
- Chicken Fricassee
- Chicken Grilled
- Chicken Marinated
- Chicken Parmigiana
- Chicken/Turkey Sausage with Onions, Peppers, and Mushrooms
- Turkey Burgers

BONELESS CHICKEN BREAST SAUTÉED

Prep time: 10 minutes
Cook time: 15 minutes

2 servings

Ingredients

2 tablespoons vegetable oil
1 whole chicken breast cut into 2 pieces without the cartilage

Instructions

1. Heat the oil in a large skillet.
2. Brown the chicken. Do not crowd. Remove the browned pieces to a plate.

Nutrient Content

Calories 198
Protein 16 gm
33% calories from Protein
Carbohydrates 0 gm
Fat 14 gm

67% calories from Fat
Cholesterol 41 mg
Sodium 46 mg
Dietary Fiber 0 gm

Adaptations for Physical Limitations

- Adjust the consistency to the swallowing ability of the client by cutting the chicken into small pieces or pureeing the food once it has completed the cooking process. Add liquid or a thickening agent if necessary.

Substitutions

- Heat vegetables or cooked potatoes in same pan.
- Use *vegetable oil spray* in place of oil.
- Add a small amount of favorite spices.

CHICKEN CUTLETS BREADED

Prep time: 15 minutes
Cook time: 15 minutes

2 servings

Ingredients

2 tablespoons vegetable oil
1 whole chicken breast cut into 2 pieces without the cartilage
$\frac{1}{3}$ cup bread crumbs either flavored or plain

1 medium egg beaten plus 1 teaspoon cold water

Instructions

1. Put bread crumbs into shallow plate.
2. Put egg into another plate near to bread crumbs plate.
3. Heat the oil in a large skillet.
4. Dip the chicken into the egg and then into the bread crumbs. Coat both sides of chicken.
5. Brown the chicken until it is no longer pink inside. Do not crowd. Remove the browned pieces to a plate.

Nutrient Content

Calories 281
Protein 21 gm
30% calories from Protein
Carbohydrates 40 gm
Fat 17 gm

56% calories from Fat
Cholesterol 135 mg
Sodium 425 mg
Dietary Fiber .5 gm

Adaptations for Physical Limitations

- Adjust the consistency to the swallowing ability of the client by cutting the chicken into small pieces or pureeing the food once it has completed the cooking process. Add liquid or a thickening agent if necessary.

Substitutions

- Heat vegetables or cooked potatoes in same pan.
- *Egg substitute* may be used in place of egg.
- Use *vegetable spray* in place of oil.
- Add various spices to bread crumbs.
- Add $\frac{1}{4}$ cup grated *Parmesan cheese* to bread crumbs.
- Use *cornflake crumbs* instead of bread crumbs for breading.
- After breading, spray each piece with vegetable oil spray and bake uncovered in a 350° oven for 25 minutes.

CHICKEN FRICASSEE

Prep time: 10 minutes
Cook time: 45 minutes

6 servings

Ingredients

1 chicken cut up into pieces
1 cup diced onion
1 cup diced celery
1 cup diced carrots
1 teaspoon garlic powder

$3/4$ teaspoon paprika
2 cups chicken broth
1 cup water
Vegetable oil spray

Instructions

1. Spray a skillet with vegetable oil spray and heat it.
2. Brown the chicken well. You may have to do this in batches.
3. Remove the chicken to a platter and keep warm.
4. Sauté the onion, celery, and carrots in the pan until they are wilted. Add small amounts of water to prevent sticking.
5. Return the chicken to the pan. Add garlic powder and paprika and broth.
6. Cook covered until chicken is done and no longer is pink inside. Add small amounts of broth or water if more liquid is needed. This will form a gravy. (This can be cooked on the stove or put into a preheated 350° oven.)

Nutrient Content

Calories 364
Protein 30 gm
34% calories from Protein
Carbohydrates 5 gm
Fat 24 gm

61% calories from Fat
Cholesterol 115 mg
Sodium 386 mg
Dietary Fiber 1 gm

Adaptations for Physical Limitations

- Adjust the consistency to the swallowing ability of the client by cutting the chicken into small pieces or pureeing the food once it has completed the cooking process. Add liquid or a thickening agent if necessary.

Substitutions

- $1/2$ cup of ***sour cream*** or $1/4$ cup of ***half and half*** may be added to the gravy after cooking.
- Chicken may be floured before browning.
- ***Green pepper*** may be added to the vegetables.
- Red pepper or hot sauce may be added to the gravy.
- 2 tablespoons of ***tomato paste*** or 1 cup of ***chopped tomatoes*** may be added to the gravy.
- Gravy may be thickened with ***flour***.
- Boneless chicken breasts may be used. Adjust the cooking time.

CHICKEN, GRILLED

Prep time: 10 minutes
Cook time: 40 minutes

4 servings

Ingredients

1 small chicken cut into parts
1 teaspoon garlic powder
1 teaspoon dried parsley

$1/2$ teaspoon paprika
Vegetable oil spray

Note: Grilling can take place on the stove in a special pan designed for this or under the broiler. You can also grill outside on a charcoal grill. DO NOT USE A CHARCOAL GRILL INSIDE.

Instructions

1. Mix the garlic, parsley, and paprika together. Rub all over the chicken.
2. Spray the grill pan or line the broiler pan with aluminum foil. Heat the grill pan or the broiler. Be sure the broiler pan will not be too close to the heat source to burn the chicken.
3. Place the chicken on the grill or the broiler.
4. Check the chicken often. Turn as it cooks. Cook for about 30 minutes or until the juices run clear.

Nutrient Content

Calories 201
Protein 35 gm
74% calories from Protein
Carbohydrates .6 gm
Fat 5 gm

25% calories from Fat
Cholesterol 115 mg
Sodium 127 mg
Dietary Fiber 0 gm

Adaptations for Physical Limitations

- Adjust the consistency to the swallowing ability of the client by cutting the chicken into small pieces or pureeing the food once it has completed the cooking process. Add liquid or a thickening agent if necessary.

Substitutions

- Any combination of herbs or spices may be used.
- Chicken breast may be used in place of chicken parts.

CHICKEN, MARINATED

Prep time: 5 minutes
2 hours refrigeration needed

Cook time: 15 minutes
2 servings

Ingredients

2 boneless chicken breasts
2 tablespoons prepared Italian salad dressing, well mixed

Note: The chicken breasts can be broiled or sautéed in a skillet. Be sure they are cooked all the way through before serving.

Instructions

1. Place the chicken breasts in a flat dish with sides.
2. Pour the salad dressing over the chicken. Cover and refrigerate at least 2 hours. May refrigerate overnight.
3. Take the chicken out and cook as preferred. Discard the marinade.

Nutrient Content

Calories 138
Protein 16 gm
49% calories from Protein
Carbohydrates 1 gm
Fat 9 gm

47% calories from Fat
Cholesterol 41 mg
Sodium 161 mg
Dietary Fiber 0 gm

Adaptations for Physical Limitations

- Adjust the consistency to the swallowing ability of the client by cutting the chicken into small pieces or pureeing the food once it has completed the cooking process. Add liquid or a thickening agent if necessary.

Substitutions

- Use chicken parts. Bake the chicken 45 minutes uncovered in a 350° oven.
- May use *fat-free salad dressing.*

CHICKEN PARMIGIANA

Prep time: 15 minutes
Cook time: 35 minutes

2 servings

Ingredients

- 2 tablespoons vegetable oil
- 1 whole chicken breast cut into 2 pieces without the cartilage
- 1/4 cup plain bread crumbs
- 1 medium egg, beaten, or egg substitute plus 1 teaspoon cold water
- 1/4 cup flour
- 1 slice of mozzarella cheese for each chicken breast (about 2 ounces total)
- 3/4 cup tomato sauce

Instructions

1. Preheat the oven to 350°.
2. Line a baking dish with aluminum foil. Spread 1/3 cup of tomato sauce in the baking dish.
3. Put bread crumbs into shallow plate.
4. Put egg into another plate near bread crumbs.
5. Put flour into a third plate.
6. Heat the oil in a large skillet.
7. Dip the chicken into the flour, then into the egg, and finally into the bread crumbs.
8. Brown the chicken. Do not crowd. Remove the browned pieces to the baking dish.
9. Pour the remaining tomato sauce over the chicken.
10. Put the cheese over each piece of chicken.
11. Bake for about 15–20 minutes until the cheese is bubbly and slightly brown.

Nutrient Content

Calories 321
Protein 31 gm
39% calories from Protein
Carbohydrates 29 gm
Fat 9 gm

24% calories from Fat
Cholesterol 151 mg
Sodium 878 mg
Dietary Fiber 2 gm

Adaptations for Physical Limitations

- Adjust the consistency to the swallowing ability of the client by cutting the chicken into small pieces or pureeing the food once it has completed the cooking process. Add liquid or a thickening agent if necessary.

Substitutions

- Add various spices to bread crumbs or used flavored bread crumbs.
- May use **vegetable spray** in place of oil.
- Add 1/4 cup grated **Parmesan cheese** to bread crumbs.
- After breading, spray each piece with vegetable oil spray and bake in a 350° oven for 25 minutes. Then top with cheese and bake.

CHICKEN/TURKEY SAUSAGE WITH ONIONS, PEPPERS, AND MUSHROOMS

Prep time: 15 minutes
Cook time: 40 minutes

3–4 servings

Ingredients

1 pound chicken or turkey sausage
1 tablespoon vegetable oil
1 cup chopped onion
$\frac{1}{2}$ cup chopped green pepper
$\frac{1}{2}$ cup sliced mushrooms

$\frac{1}{4}$ teaspoon chopped parsley
$\frac{1}{2}$ teaspoon chopped basil
$\frac{1}{2}$ teaspoon chopped oregano
$1\frac{1}{2}$ cup tomato sauce

Instructions

1. Cut the sausage into bite-size pieces.
2. Heat the oil in a skillet.
3. Brown the sausage about 10 minutes.
4. Add the onion, green pepper, and mushroom. Cook about 10 minutes.
5. Add the spices and tomato sauce. Cook additional 10–15 minutes or until the meat is cooked thoroughly.

Nutrient Content

Calories 275
Protein 18 gm
23% calories from Protein
Carbohydrates gm
Fat 20 gm

58% calories from Fat
Cholesterol 0 mg
Sodium 1557 mg
Dietary Fiber 2 gm

Adaptations for Physical Limitations

- Adjust the consistency to the swallowing ability of the client by cutting the sausage into small pieces or pureeing the food once it has completed the cooking process. Add liquid or a thickening agent if necessary.

Substitutions

- Add **Parmesan cheese** when serving.
- Add hot red pepper flakes when serving.
- Use **tomato sauce with no added salt.**
- Use **veal, lamb,** or **pork sausage.**

TURKEY BURGERS

Prep time: 10 minutes
Cook time: 15–20 minutes

4 servings

Ingredients

1 pound ground turkey (97% lean, no skin)
4 large egg whites
½ teaspoon garlic powder
½ teaspoon dried parsley
¼ teaspoon black pepper
½ cup diced celery
½ cup diced onion
Vegetable oil spray

Instructions

1. Mix all ingredients thoroughly.
2. Form into 5-ounce patties.
3. Grill until each side is brown and center is cooked.

Nutrient Content

Calories 150
Protein 31 gm
82% calories from Protein
Carbohydrates 3 gm
Fat 2 gm
11% calories from Fat
Cholesterol 55 mg
Sodium 144 mg
Dietary Fiber .6 gm

Adaptations for Physical Limitations

- Adjust the consistency to the swallowing ability of the client by cutting the turkey into small pieces or pureeing the food once it has completed the cooking process. Add liquid or a thickening agent if necessary.

Substitutions

- Use 2 large *eggs* in place of 4 egg whites.
- Add 1 teaspoon *soy sauce* if desired.
- Add *salt* to taste if desired.
- Omit the *onions* as needed.
- Melt *cheese* on top of burger.
- Serve with lettuce and tomato slices.
- Serve on hamburger *bun*.

Introduction for Fish

The prevalence of fish in the American diet has increased within the last 10 years due to:

- The identification of the positive health benefits of eating fish.
- The increasing variety of fish available in most parts of the country
- The availability of books and teachers to share the cooking methods with the homemaker.
- The fact that fish does not take very long to cook.

Many people, however, do not like fish. They are not comfortable with the smell, taste, or preparation of it. Some people are allergic to shellfish. Although most people would benefit from eating fish, if your clients do not include fish in their diet, you can encourage them to taste some mild fish, but you may not overcome this preference.

Some people have ethnic or religious preferences for and against certain fish. Some people eat certain fish at certain times of the year and to mark certain occasions. Respect these habits and include these in your meal planning.

When preparing fish, the following seasonings can help you to vary the taste:

Lemon	Parsley
Paprika	Garlic
Onion	Cilantro
Ginger	Bay leaf (remove from the dish before eating)
Fennel	Dill
Marjoram	Thyme

Fish is perishable. It should always be kept in the refrigerator until it is ready to be cooked. It should be defrosted in the refrigerator, not on the counter, and should not be refrozen. Most fish is eaten completely cooked. Recently, however, some types of fish are eaten "rare." This practice should be discussed with your supervisor and/or a nutritionist. Raw fish, eaten by some cultures, is never frozen and eaten very close to the time the fish is caught. If your client likes to eat raw fish, discuss with your supervisor the best way to obtain the most appropriate fish for this purpose.

Recipes included in this section of this chapter:

- Baked Fish
- Creole Fish
- Pan-Fried Fish

BAKED FISH

Prep time: 10 minutes
Cook time: 15 minutes

2 servings

Ingredients

2 pieces of fish, either steaks or fillets (about 4–6 ounces each)
¼ cup water
¼ teaspoon dill

1 teaspoon butter
1–2 teaspoons lemon juice
½ teaspoon black pepper

Instructions

1. Preheat the oven to 350°.
2. Put the fish in an ovenproof dish. Do not crowd.
3. Put water in the dish.
4. Put the dill and butter on the fish. (If you do not use butter, spray the fish with vegetable oil spray.)
5. Bake in the oven, uncovered for 10 to 15 minutes or until the fish is lightly browned.
6. Season with pepper and lemon juice.

Nutrient Content

Calories 167
Protein 31 gm
77% calories from Protein
Carbohydrates 0 gm
Fat 4 gm

22% calories from Fat
Cholesterol 91 mg
Sodium 149 mg
Dietary Fiber 0 gm

Adaptations for Physical Limitations

- Adjust the consistency to the swallowing ability of the client by chopping or flaking the fish with a fork or pureeing the fish once it has completed the cooking process. Add liquid or a thickening agent if necessary.

Substitutions

- Add cooked vegetable to the cooking dish.
- Add hot red pepper flakes when serving.
- *Vegetable spray* may be used in place of butter.
- Fish could be breaded in *bread crumbs* before baking. Spray the pan with vegetable oil spray. Do not put the water in the pan.

CREOLE FISH

Prep time: 15 minutes
Cook time: 15–25 minutes

2–3 servings

Ingredients

12 ounces cleaned whitefish, without head, or fillets or steaks
1 15-ounce can no-salt stewed tomatoes cut into small pieces
1/8 cup chopped onion
1/8 cup chopped green pepper

1/4 teaspoon basil
1/4 teaspoon thyme
1/4 teaspoon chopped parsley
Vegetable oil spray
1–2 teaspoons lemon juice

Instructions

1. Preheat the oven to 350°.
2. Line a baking dish with aluminum foil. Spray foil with cooking oil spray.
3. Put the fish in an ovenproof dish. Do not crowd.
4. Pour the tomatoes around the fish.
5. Add the green pepper, onions, basil, thyme, and parsley.
6. Bake in the oven covered for 10–15 minutes or until the fish is cooked.
7. Season with lemon juice.

Nutrient Content

Calories 162
Protein 32gm
83% calories from Protein
Carbohydrates 2 gm
Fat 2 gm

12% calories from Fat
Cholesterol 82 mg
Sodium 141 mg
Dietary Fiber .5 gm

Adaptations for Physical Limitations

- Adjust the consistency to the swallowing ability of the client by chopping or flaking the fish with a fork or pureeing the fish once it has completed the cooking process. Add liquid or a thickening agent if necessary.

Substitutions

- Add cooked *vegetable* to the cooking dish.
- Add hot red pepper flakes when serving.

PAN-FRIED FISH

Prep time: 10 minutes
Cook time: 15 minutes

2 servings

Ingredients

12-ounce fillet or fish steaks or 1 whole fish cleaned, without head

Vegetable oil spray
1–2 tablespoon lemon juice

Instructions

1. Spray the skillet with vegetable oil spray.
2. Heat the skillet.
3. Place the fish in it and adjust the heat so it doesn't burn. Cook until the fish is lightly browned.
4. Turn and cook the second side.
5. Add lemon juice.

Nutrient Content

Calories 156
Protein 31 gm
82% calories from Protein
Carbohydrates 3 gm
Fat 2 gm

12% calories from Fat
Cholesterol 78 mg
Sodium 132 mg
Dietary Fiber 0 gm

Adaptations for Physical Limitations

- Adjust the consistency to the swallowing ability of the client by chopping or flaking the fish with a fork or pureeing the fish once it has completed the cooking process. Add liquid or a thickening agent if necessary.

Substitutions

- Vary the spices on the fish after cooking.
- Add *stewed tomatoes* after cooking.
- Fish could be breaded in *flour and/or bread crumbs* before cooking.

Introduction for Meatless

Meatless meals are a very useful and nutritionally sound way to introduce variety into a diet. Although it is a challenge, nutritional requirements can be met.

Meatless entrees have several positive features:

- They can usually be prepared in advance.
- Ingredients can be changed to accommodate varied tastes and availability of ingredients.
- Meals are easily frozen.
- Most dishes can be served either as main course or an accompaniment to another dish.
- Meatless dishes are easy on the budget.

Pasta dishes can be varied with the use of various combinations of seasonings. The following should be considered when varying recipes:

Basil   Oregano
Tomato   Onion
Garlic   Green pepper
Red pepper   Pine nuts
Low-fat/low-sodium cheese

Recipes included in this section of this chapter:

- Eggplant Parmigiana (Low Fat)
- Macaroni and Cheese
- Pasta Primavera
- Quick Tomato Sauce
- Stuffed Shells

EGGPLANT PARMIGIANA (LOW FAT)

Prep time: 35 minutes
Cook time: 40 minutes

4 servings

Ingredients

1 eggplant cut into $\frac{1}{2}$-inch slices
$1\frac{1}{2}$ cups tomato and herb pasta sauce
$\frac{1}{2}$ teaspoon parsley
$\frac{1}{2}$ cup bread crumbs

$\frac{1}{2}$ cup Parmesan cheese grated
8 ounces sliced nonfat mozzarella cheese
Vegetable oil spray

Instructions

1. Heat the oven to 325°.
2. Spray each piece of eggplant with vegetable oil spray and dip into bread crumbs.
3. Place on large cookie sheet.
4. Bake in the oven 15 minutes. Turn each piece over. Bake another 12 minutes or until they are brown.
5. Arrange the eggplant into a baking dish. You can put two slices on top of each other if you put sauce and cheese between them.
6. Spray aluminum foil with vegetable oil spray and cover the eggplant with sprayed side down.
7. Bake for 25 minutes.
8. Uncover and bake another 15 minutes or until cheese is brown and bubbly.
9. Cool 10 minutes before slicing.

Nutrient Content

Calories 258
Protein 28 gm
42% calories from Protein
Carbohydrates 27 gm
Fat 5 gm

16% calories from Fat
Cholesterol 20 mg
Sodium 1045 mg
Dietary Fiber 5 gm

Adaptations for Physical Limitations

- Adjust to client's ability to swallow by cutting the eggplant into small pieces, pureeing the food once it has completed the cooking process. Add liquid or thickening agent if necessary.

Substitutions

- Add cayenne pepper to taste.
- Vary the *cheeses* used.
- Put *mushrooms or zucchini* into the tomato sauce before cooking.
- Serve with *pasta*.

MACARONI AND CHEESE

Prep time: 10 minutes
Cook time: 45 minutes

4 servings

Ingredients

½ pound elbow macaroni or small shells
3 tablespoons butter
3 tablespoons flour

3 cups whole milk
1 ounce crushed tomatoes
2¼ cups grated cheddar cheese

Instructions

1. Preheat the oven to 350°.
2. Heat water and cook the macaroni. Drain. Do not rinse.
3. Melt the butter in a saucepan.
4. When the butter is bubbling, add the flour and continue to stir. Slowly add the milk, stirring all the time. When all the milk is added, the sauce should be lump free.
5. Stir in the cheddar cheese. Add the tomatoes.
6. Mix the macaroni and the sauce together and place it in a casserole.
7. Bake until the top is brown and the casserole is hot.

Nutrient Content

Calories 538
Protein 26 gm
19% calories from Protein
Carbohydrates 21 gm
Fat 40 gm

66% calories from Fat
Cholesterol 127 mg
Sodium 728 mg
Dietary Fiber 0 gm

Adaptations for Physical Limitations

- Adjust the consistency to the swallowing ability of the client by cutting the macaroni into small pieces. It may be mashed.

Substitutions

- Other *cheeses* may be used with or instead of the cheddar, such as Swiss, Monterey Jack, flavored cheddar, Asiago.
- May use all *skim milk* or *low-fat milk,* but not evaporated, sweetened, or chocolate milk.

PASTA PRIMAVERA

Prep time: 20 minutes
Cook time: 20 minutes

4 servings

Ingredients

1 cup broccoli florets
1 cup fresh mushrooms, cleaned and cut in half
½ red pepper, sliced in strips
1 tablespoon chopped chives
½ cup low-fat sour cream
¼ cup sliced carrots (coin shaped)
4 ounces shredded cheddar cheese
6 ounces spaghetti

Instructions

1. Prepare spaghetti and keep warm.
2. Steam broccoli, mushrooms, and pepper until crisp but tender.
3. Toss in chives.
4. Combine sour cream, carrots, and half of the cheese.
5. Toss with spaghetti.
6. Arrange on serving platter.
7. Top with vegetable mixture.
8. Sprinkle with remaining cheese.

Nutrient Content

Calories 217
Protein 8 gm
15% calories from Protein
Carbohydrates 38 gm
Fat 3 gm

14% calories from Fat
Cholesterol 9 mg
Sodium 43 mg
Dietary Fiber 2 gm

Adaptations for Physical Limitations

- Adjust the consistency to the swallowing ability of the client by chopping vegetables. The pasta and vegetables may be mashed.

Substitutions

- Any fresh or frozen *vegetable* can be added. Adjust cooking times.
- Any pasta can be substituted in place of spaghetti.
- Add hot pepper.

QUICK TOMATO SAUCE

Prep time: 10 minutes
Cook time: 25 minutes

4 servings

Ingredients

1 28-ounce can of crushed tomatoes
1 teaspoon oregano
1 teaspoon garlic powder

1 teaspoon dried parsley
$\frac{1}{2}$ teaspoon dried basil
2 teaspoons tomato paste

Instructions

1. Combine all ingredients in a pot.
2. Cook until the sauce is thickened.

Nutrient Content

Calories 68
Protein 4 gm
24% calories from Protein
Carbohydrates 12 gm
Fat 0 gm

1% calories from Fat
Cholesterol 0 mg
Sodium 3 mg
Dietary Fiber 0 gm

Adaptations for Physical Limitations

- None

Substitutions

- Add *sausage* or *cooked chopped meat*. Small pieces of cooked *ham* or *salami* may also be used.
- *Meatballs* may be added.

STUFFED SHELLS

Prep time: 35 minutes
Cook time: 45 minutes

Storage: In refrigerator
6 servings

Ingredients

½ pound of large pasta shells for stuffing
½ pound ricotta cheese
1 medium egg
½ teaspoon oregano
½ teaspoon parsley

½ teaspoon basil
½ teaspoon garlic powder
½ pound mozzarella cheese
1½ cups tomato sauce
½ cup grated Parmesan cheese

Instructions

1. Bring a large pot of water to a boil. Put the noodles into the pot and cook according to directions. Drain well.
2. Preheat oven to 325°.
3. Mix the ricotta cheese, oregano, parsley, basil, and garlic.
4. Put ⅓ of tomato sauce in bottom of baking dish at least 2 inches deep.
5. Stuff each shell with the cheese mixture. Do not put too much in each shell.
6. Place each shell in the baking dish pasta side down and cheese side up.
7. Spray aluminum foil with vegetable spray and cover the shells with sprayed side down.
8. Bake for 30 minutes.
9. Uncover and bake another 15 minutes or until cheese is brown and bubbly.
10. Cool 10 minutes before serving.

Nutrient Content

Calories 392
Protein 22 gm
24% calories from Protein
Carbohydrates 36 gm
Fat 16 gm

39% calories from Fat
Cholesterol 70 mg
Sodium 752 mg
Dietary Fiber 2 gm

Adaptations for Physical Limitations

- Adjust to client's ability to swallow by cutting shells into small pieces.

Substitutions

- Add cayenne pepper to taste.
- Vary the *cheeses* used
- Use *low-fat* or *low-salt cheeses* in place of regular.
- Put mushrooms or zucchini into the tomato sauce before cooking.
- Use *egg substitute* instead of egg.

CHAPTER 16
Recipes for Vegetables

Introduction

Although there are many jokes about eating vegetables and often eating them was seen as a punishment rather than an activity to be enjoyed, vegetables have gained increased importance in our diets for several reasons:

- As a result of improved packing and travel arrangements, vegetables from all parts of the world can reach almost any supermarket. Therefore, all vegetables can be enjoyed throughout the year rather than waiting for them to be available locally.
- Scientific evidence has indicated that vegetables contribute important elements to our diet and greatly improve overall health.
- Vegetables are a good way to decrease calories during and in between meals and increase the natural intake of vitamins, fiber, and micronutrients.
- Vegetables can be part of the meal as an accompaniment to the entrée, used as part of the entrée, put into the salad, or eaten in-between meals as a snack.

Vegetables are usually cooked according to the preference of the eater. Some people like them well cooked and soft, while others enjoy them partially cooked and crispy. Some people salt the cooking water; others do not. Some people enjoy vegetables with sauce; others like them plain with some butter or lemon juice. Some people will eat the skin; others will not. Discuss with your clients his or her preference and adhere to it.

Vegetables can be cooked by several methods and often as part of another dish. For example, carrots can be cooked on top of the stove in a little bit of water, in the microwave, or as part of a stew. You are encouraged to experiment and discuss with your client his individual preferences.

- Always wash the vegetable before cooking them.
- When cutting vegetables, try to have the pieces about the same size so they will cook at the same rate.
- Usually root vegetables, such as carrots, turnips, and parsnips will be peeled before cooking.
- Similar vegetables can be cooked by similar methods.

Try cooking these vegetables separately or together and then serve them mixed together for variety.

Brussels sprouts and celery
Carrot slices and lima beans
Carrots and celery
Carrots and green beans
Carrots and green peas
Cauliflower and green peas
Celery and mushrooms
Corn and green lima beans
Corn and green peas
Mushrooms and green peas
Okra and tomatoes
Onions and green peas
Squash, tomatoes, and onions
Tomatoes and zucchini

Recipes included in this chapter:

- Baked Acorn Squash
- Broccoli, Steamed
- Carrots (Basic)
- Grated Zucchini
- Green Beans Sauté
- Vegetables, Canned
- Vegetables, Frozen

BAKED ACORN SQUASH

Prep time: 10 minutes
Cook time: 55 minutes

4 servings

Ingredients

2 acorn squash
¼ cup butter

¼ cup packed light brown sugar
½ teaspoon ground cinnamon

Instructions

1. Preheat oven to 350°.
2. Cut squash in half lengthwise and remove seeds.
3. Place in baking pan, cut side down. Bake for 35 minutes or until tender.
4. Remove from oven. Turn cut side up in baking pan.
5. Dot with butter.
6. Mix brown sugar and cinnamon together. Sprinkle on top.
7. Put back in oven and bake 20 minutes longer.
8. Scoop out flesh and serve.

Nutrient Content

Calories 212
Protein 1 gm
2% calories from Protein
Carbohydrates 29 gm
Fat 12 gm

47% calories from Fat
Cholesterol 31 mg
Sodium 127 mg
Dietary Fiber 5 gm

Adaptations for Physical Limitations

- Adjust the consistency to the swallowing ability of the client by cutting the squash into small pieces or pureeing the food once it has completed the cooking process. Add liquid or a thickening agent if necessary.

Substitutions

- May use *margarine* in place of butter.
- Omit *butter* and add ½ cup *orange juice* to pan before baking.
- Use 2 tablespoons *honey* instead of brown sugar.

BROCCOLI, STEAMED

Prep time: 5 minutes
Cook time: 5 minutes

1 serving

Ingredients

3 broccoli spears

3 tablespoon water

Instructions

1. Place washed broccoli on a microwavable dish.
2. Pour water in the dish and cover with plastic wrap.
3. Microwave about 5 minutes depending on the strength of the microwave and the way the client likes the vegetables.

Nutrient Content

Calories 30
Protein 3 gm
36% calories from Protein
Carbohydrates 5 gm
Fat 0 gm

5% calories from Fat
Cholesterol 0 mg
Sodium 31 mg
Dietary Fiber 0 gm

Adaptations for Physical Limitations

- Adjust the consistency to the swallowing ability of the client by cutting the broccoli into small pieces or pureeing the food once it has completed the cooking process. Add liquid or a thickening agent if necessary.

Substitutions

- Substitute any vegetable or combination of vegetables.
- Add 1 teaspoon **butter**.
- Serve with lemon juice or lemon wedge.

CARROTS (BASIC)

Prep time: 10 minutes
Cook time: 15 minutes

4 servings

Ingredients

1 pound carrots, peeled and cut into ¼-inch circles
3 tablespoons unsalted butter
½ teaspoon sugar
1½ cups water
1 tablespoon chopped parsley

Instructions

1. In medium saucepan, add carrots, butter, sugar, water, and parsley.
2. Cook uncovered over medium heat until carrots are tender and water has almost evaporated, about 15 minutes.
3. Serve immediately.

Nutrient Content

Calories 127
Protein 1 gm
4% calories from Protein
Carbohydrates 12 gm
Fat 9 gm

60% calories from Fat
Cholesterol 23 mg
Sodium 44 mg
Dietary Fiber 3 gm

Adaptations for Physical Limitations

- Adjust the consistency to the swallowing ability of the client by cutting the carrots into small pieces or pureeing the food once it has completed the cooking process. Add liquid or a thickening agent if necessary.

Substitutions

- Omit *sugar*.
- Add 1 teaspoon of *honey* in place of sugar.

GRATED ZUCCHINI

Prep time: 5 minutes
Cook time: 10 minutes

4 servings

Ingredients

2 tablespoons unsalted butter
1 clove garlic, peeled and diced
3 medium zucchini, washed, unpeeled, and grated

1/4 teaspoon nutmeg

Instructions

1. In large pan, melt the butter and sauté garlic over medium heat for 3–4 minutes. Do not brown.
2. Add the zucchini. Mix well.
3. Cook until tender. May need to add water to cooking process.
4. Add nutmeg, mix.

Nutrient Content

Calories 73
Protein 2 gm
9% calories from Protein
Carbohydrates 5 gm
Fat 6 gm

68% calories from Fat
Cholesterol 16 mg
Sodium 5 mg
Dietary Fiber 2 gm

Adaptations for Physical Limitations

- Adjust the consistency to the swallowing ability of the client by cutting the zucchini into small pieces or pureeing the food once it has completed the cooking process. Add liquid or a thickening agent if necessary.

Substitutions

- May use *yellow squash* in place of zucchini.
- May use 1/4 teaspoon garlic powder in place of clove.
- May use *margarine* in place of butter.
- May use *vegetable oil spray* instead of butter.
- May add *cheese* at time of serving.

GREEN BEANS SAUTÉ

Prep time: 5 minutes
Cook time: 5 minutes

2 servings

Ingredients

½ pound green beans

1 tablespoon unsalted butter

Instructions

1. Rinse the green beans. Cook in boiling water for 3–4 minutes.
2. Drain well.
3. Melt the butter in frying pan, add the cooked beans.
4. Drizzle melted butter over beans, mix well.
4. Cook until hot.

Nutrient Content

Calories 86
Protein 2 gm
9% calories from Protein
Carbohydrates 8 gm
Fat 6 gm

56% calories from Fat
Cholesterol 16 mg
Sodium 8 mg
Dietary Fiber 4 gm

Adaptations for Physical Limitations

- Adjust the consistency to the swallowing ability of the client by cutting the green beans into small pieces or pureeing the food once it has completed the cooking process. Add liquid or a thickening agent if necessary.

Substitutions

- Add *salt* and pepper to taste.
- Add roasted slivered *almonds*.
- Use *vegetable oil spray* instead of butter.
- Add 2 tablespoons chopped *onion* to green beans as they sauté.

VEGETABLES, CANNED

Prep time: 5 minutes
Cook time: 5 minutes

2 servings

Ingredients

1 8-ounce can of mixed vegetables

½ cup water

Instructions

1. Open can of mixed vegetables.
2. Rinse and drain.
3. In pan heat water until boiling.
4. Add vegetables, heat thoroughly about 5 minutes

Nutrient Content

Calories 38
Protein 2 gm
21% calories from Protein
Carbohydrates 8 gm
Fat 0 gm

0% calories from Fat
Cholesterol 0 mg
Sodium 123 mg
Dietary Fiber 2 gm

Adaptations for Physical Limitations

- Adjust the consistency to the swallowing ability of the client by pureeing the food once it has completed the cooking process. Add liquid or a thickening agent if necessary.

Substitutions

- Any seasonings or spices can be added during or after cooking.
- Serve with entrées or salads.

VEGETABLES, FROZEN

Prep time: None
Cook time: 10 minutes

2 servings

Ingredients

1 cup frozen mixed vegetables

¼ cup water

Instructions

1. Place frozen vegetables and water in pot.
2. Cover and boil over medium heat for 7–10 minutes or until desired tenderness.
3. Drain.
4. Serve.

Nutrient Content

Calories 30
Protein 1 gm
15% calories from Protein
Carbohydrates 7 gm
Fat 0 gm

9% calories from Fat
Cholesterol 0 mg
Sodium 11 mg
Dietary Fiber 0 gm

Adaptations for Physical Limitations

- Adjust the consistency to the swallowing ability of the client by pureeing the food once it has completed the cooking process. Add liquid or a thickening agent if necessary.

Substitutions

- Any variety of **vegetables** can be mixed together.
- Add **margarine** or **butter** prior to serving.
- Any seasonings can be added after or during cooking.

CHAPTER 17

Recipes for Rice, Potato, and Pasta

Introduction

Rice, potatoes, and pasta are common accompaniments to a balanced meal. They provide texture, taste, and a vehicle for other nutrients such as vegetables and sometimes protein. Every culture has a favorite food from this group. Asian countries serve a great deal of rice, while Italy serves great deal of pasta.

When discussing this food group with clients, it is wise to find out the following:

- Do they eat pasta, rice, or potatoes at every meal?
- Do they eat long-grain, short-grain, or medium-grain rice?
- Do they eat brown or white rice?
- Do they make their own pasta or buy it fresh or dry?
- How much of each is considered an adult portion?

Rice, pasta, and potatoes are often left over from a meal. Store uneaten portions covered in the refrigerator, and add vegetables or protein to them for a second meal.

You will be able to vary the taste of the rice by varying the cooking liquid to include all clear broths and gravies. Depending on the consistency of the rice the client likes, you may have to add more liquid to the recipes.

Recipes included in this chapter:

Rice

- Brown Rice
- Fried Rice Chinese Style
- Rice and Beans

- Rice Indian Style
- Rice Mexican Style
- Rice Pilaf
- Rice with Lentils

Potato

- Baked Potato (Oven and Microwave)
- Boiled Potato
- Home Fried Potatoes
- Mashed Potatoes
- Potato Croquettes
- Rosemary Garlic Sweet Potatoes
- Roasted Potatoes

Pasta

- Pasta with Beans
- Pasta with Butter
- Pasta with Garlic and Oil
- Pasta with Herbs and Cheese
- Pasta with Quick Tomato Sauce

Other Grains

- Barley with Mushrooms
- Grits Casserole
- Quinoa
- Taboulleh

Additional Pasta Recipes Located in Chapter 15, Entrees, Meatless Section

- Macaroni and Cheese
- Pasta Primavera
- Stuffed Shells

BROWN RICE

Prep time: 2 minutes
Cook time: 25 minutes

4 servings

Ingredients

1 cup brown long-grain rice

2 cups water

Instructions

1. Bring water to a boil in a covered saucepan.
2. Put rice into water. Cover and bring back to a boil.
3. Cook 20 minutes covered at a low boil until water has been absorbed and rice is tender. You may have to add additional water and cook a little longer.

Nutrient Content

Calories 150
Protein 3 gm
8% calories from Protein
Carbohydrates 32 gm
Fat 1 gm

6% calories from Fat
Cholesterol 0 mg
Sodium 4 mg
Dietary Fiber 1 gm

Adaptations for Physical Limitations

- Adjust the consistency to the swallowing ability of the client by mashing the rice. May be pureed if needed in blender; add additional liquid to get to desired consistency.

Substitutions

- Use any clear **broth** as liquid. May be mixed with water.
- Use defatted **chicken** or **turkey gravy**. Add enough water to make 2 cups.

FRIED RICE CHINESE STYLE

Prep time: 5 minutes
Cook time: 10 minutes

4 servings

Ingredients

2 cups white long-grain rice, cooked and cooled
1 clove minced garlic
2 tablespoons minced green onion
2 tablespoons soy sauce
1 egg beaten
1 tablespoon canola oil

Instructions

1. Heat the oil in a large frying pan.
2. Add the garlic and sauté 1 minute.
3. Add the rice. Break any lumps. Heat thoroughly. If the rice sticks, add a tablespoon of water.
4. Make a hole in the center of the rice. Add the egg into the hole and beat it and the rice together so that the scrambled egg and the rice are all together.
5. Add the soy sauce.
6. Sprinkle the green onions on top of the rice as you serve it.

Nutrient Content

Calories 169
Protein 4 gm
11% calories from Protein
Carbohydrates 27 gm
Fat 5 gm
25% calories from Fat
Cholesterol 47 mg
Sodium 474 mg
Dietary Fiber 0 gm

Adaptations for Physical Limitations

- Adjust the consistency to the swallowing ability of the client by mashing the rice and cutting the vegetables into small pieces.

Substitutions

- Add any cooked **meat, fish** or **poultry** cut into small pieces.
- Add $\frac{1}{2}$ cup **bean sprouts,** $\frac{1}{2}$ cup cooked **peas,** $\frac{1}{2}$ cup sliced **water chestnuts,** or $\frac{1}{2}$ cup cooked **mushrooms.**
- Use **low-salt soy sauce.**
- Use **vegetable oil spray** instead of oil.
- May eat 2 servings as main course of a meal.

RICE AND BEANS

Prep time: 10 minutes
Cook time: 25 minutes

4 servings

Ingredients

1 tablespoon canola oil
1 cup minced onion
2 tablespoons minced garlic

1 cup long-grain rice
1½ cups cooked black beans
2 cups chicken broth

Instructions

1. Heat oil in saucepan.
2. Cook onions and garlic until tender.
3. Stir in the rice and add the liquid. Bring to a boil.
4. Stir in the beans. Cover and cook until all liquid has been absorbed.

Nutrient Content

Calories 196
Protein 8 gm
16% from Protein
Carbohydrates 30 gm
Fat 5 gm

24% calories from Fat
Cholesterol 0 mg
Sodium 801 mg
Dietary Fiber 6 gm

Adaptations for Physical Limitations

- Adjust the consistency to the swallowing ability of the client by mashing the rice and beans.

Substitutions

- Add ½ cup chopped **canned tomatoes.**
- Add red pepper flakes or chili peppers before serving.
- Use **vegetable oil spray** instead of oil.
- Use **low-sodium chicken broth.**

RICE INDIAN STYLE

Prep time: 10 minutes
Cook time: 25 minutes

4 servings

Ingredients

1 teaspoon canola oil
1 cup sliced onion
1 bay leaf
1 teaspoon cardamom

1 cup basmati rice
$1/4$ teaspoon cinnamon
$1/4$ teaspoon ground ginger
2 cups chicken broth

Instructions

1. Heat the oil in a saucepan.
2. Cook the onions, bay leaf, and cardamom until the onions are clear.
3. Add the rice and stir so all the spices are mixed well.
4. Add the ginger, cinnamon, and the stock.
5. Cover and cook until the liquid is absorbed.
6. Remove the bay leaf before serving.

Nutrient Content

Calories 219
Protein 4 gm
9% calories from Protein
Carbohydrates 42 gm
Fat 2 gm

10% calories from Fat
Cholesterol 0 mg
Sodium 501 mg
Dietary Fiber 2 gm

Adaptations for Physical Limitations

- Adjust the consistency to the swallowing ability of the client by mashing the rice.

Substitutions

- Add $1/4$ teaspoon of saffron to the stock.
- Serve with sliced ***chicken*** or cooked ***beef***.

RICE MEXICAN STYLE

Prep time: 10 minutes
Cook time: 35 minutes

4 servings

Ingredients

1 teaspoon minced garlic
1 cup minced onion
½ cup minced green pepper
1 cup cooked crushed tomatoes

½ teaspoon paprika
1 cup long-grain rice
2 cups chicken broth
Vegetable oil spray

Instructions

1. Spray a saucepan with vegetable oil spray.
2. Heat the sauce pan and cook the onions and garlic until the onions are clear.
3. Add the rice and stir until the rice becomes toasted and brown.
4. Add the green pepper, tomatoes, and chicken broth. Cover and cook until the liquid is absorbed.
5. Add the paprika and serve.

Nutrient Content

Calories 214
Protein 5 gm
10% calories from Protein
Carbohydrates 44 gm
Fat 1 gm

6% calories from Fat
Cholesterol 0 mg
Sodium 614 mg
Dietary Fiber 2 gm

Adaptations for Physical Limitations

- Adjust the consistency to the swallowing ability of the client by mashing the rice.

Substitutions

- Add red pepper flakes before serving.

RICE PILAF

Prep time: 8 minutes
Cook time: 30 minutes

4 servings

Ingredients

1 tablespoon canola oil
1/3 cup diced onion
1 cup long-grain rice
2 cups nonfat/low-sodium chicken broth

Instructions

1. Heat the oil in a saucepan.
2. Cook the onions until they are clear.
3. Add the rice and stir until it is slightly brown and toasted.
4. Add the chicken stock. Cover and cook until liquid is absorbed.

Nutrient Content

Calories 190
Protein 4 gm
9% calories from Protein
Carbohydrates 34 gm
Fat 4 gm
17% calories from Fat
Cholesterol 0 mg
Sodium 30 mg
Dietary Fiber 0 gm

Adaptations for Physical Limitations

- Adjust the consistency to the swallowing ability of the client by mashing the rice.

Substitutions

- Vary the cooking liquid to include **beef stock** or **vegetable stock.**
- Use **vegetable oil spray** instead of oil.

RICE WITH LENTILS

Prep time: 5 minutes
Cook time: 45 minutes

4 servings

Ingredients

2½ cups nonfat/low-sodium chicken broth
1 cup long-grain rice
½ cup raw lentils

1 bay leaf
¼ cup diced onion

Instructions

1. Heat the chicken stock in a saucepan.
2. Add the rest of the ingredients.
3. Cook covered until the liquid is absorbed.
4. Remove the bay leaf before serving.

Nutrient Content

Calories 241
Protein 11 gm
19% calories from Protein
Carbohydrates 47 gm
Fat 0 gm

1% calories from Fat
Cholesterol 0 mg
Sodium 40 mg
Dietary Fiber 8 gm

Adaptations for Physical Limitations

- Adjust the consistency to the swallowing ability of the client by mashing the rice and lentils.

Substitutions

- Omit the onions.

BAKED POTATO (OVEN AND MICROWAVE)

Prep time: 2 minutes
Cook time: 45 minutes in the oven;
6 minutes in the microwave

1 serving

Ingredients

1 medium-size baking potato

1 teaspoon unsalted butter

Instructions

Oven method of cooking

1. Place washed potato in a 350° oven.
2. Let bake about 45 minutes or until the potato is soft.
3. Slice open and put butter on it.

Microwave method of cooking

1. Place washed potato in microwave for 5 minutes.
2. Test to see that it is soft. If not, put it back for another 30 seconds.
3. Slice open and put butter on it.

Nutrient Content

Calories 132
Protein 3 gm
8% calories from Protein
Carbohydrates 22 gm
Fat 4 gm

28% calories from Fat
Cholesterol 11 mg
Sodium 8 mg
Dietary Fiber 2 gm

Adaptations for Physical Limitations

- Adjust the consistency to the swallowing ability of the client by mashing the potato and cutting the skin into small pieces.

Substitutions

- Serve with any type of *cheese* on top of opened potato.
- Serve with *yogurt* or *sour cream.*
- Add chopped onions, dill, chives, or parsley.

BOILED POTATO

Prep time: 2 minutes
Cook time: 15 minutes

1 serving

Ingredients

1 medium potato, peeled or not peeled, washed

Water to cover the potato
1 teaspoon unsalted butter

Instructions

1. Put potato into the cold water and bring to a boil.
2. Cook covered until potato is soft and can be poked easily with a fork.
3. Drain. May be peeled or not
4. Toss with a teaspoon of butter.

Nutrient Content

Calories 132
Protein 3 gm
8% calories from Protein
Carbohydrates 22 gm
Fat 4 gm

28% calories from Fat
Cholesterol 11 mg
Sodium 8 mg
Dietary Fiber 2 gm

Adaptations for Physical Limitations

- Adjust the consistency to the swallowing ability of the client by mashing the potato.

Substitutions

- Add chopped onions, dill, chives, or parsley.
- Vary the spices

HOME FRIED POTATOES

Prep time: 2 minutes
Cook time: 20 minutes

1 serving

Ingredients

1 medium potato, peeled or not peeled
Water to cover the potato

2 tablespoons vegetable oil

Instructions

1. Put potato into the cold water to cover potato and bring to a boil.
2. Cook covered until potato is soft and can be poked easily with a fork.
3. Drain. May be peeled or not. (This may be done up to one day in advance.)
4. Heat the oil in a frying pan.
5. Slice the potato into thin slices.
6. Fry until brown; turn and brown second side.
7. Put fried potatoes on a paper towel and drain.

Nutrient Content

Calories 336
Protein 3 gm
3% calories from Protein
Carbohydrates 22 gm
Fat 28 gm

72% calories from Fat
Cholesterol 0 mg
Sodium 7 mg
Dietary Fiber 2 gm

Adaptations for Physical Limitations

- Adjust the consistency to the swallowing ability of the client by cutting the potatoes into small pieces.

Substitutions

- Fry *onions* with the potatoes.
- Add sliced or diced *peppers*.

MASHED POTATOES

Prep time: 5 minutes
Cook time: 15 minutes

1 serving

Ingredients

1 medium potato cut into slices, peeled or not peeled
Water to cover the potato

1 teaspoon unsalted butter
2 tablespoons milk

Instructions

1. Put potato into the cold water to barely cover and bring to a boil.
2. Cook covered until potato is soft and can be poked easily with a fork and the water is absorbed.
3. Use a potato masher or a fork to mash the potato. (Some people like chunks; others do not.)
4. Add the butter and milk. You may have to add more or less milk to achieve the consistency the client likes.

Nutrient Content

Calories 151
Protein 4 gm
9% calories from Protein
Carbohydrates 23 gm
Fat 5 gm

30% calories from Fat
Cholesterol 15 mg
Sodium 23 mg
Dietary Fiber 2 gm

Adaptations for Physical Limitations

- Adjust the consistency to the swallowing ability of the client by mashing potato and adding enough milk for the right consistency.

Substitutions

- Add various spices.
- Sprinkle with $1/4$ teaspoon paprika and put under the broiler for 5 minutes.
- Use any *milk,* except chocolate milk.
- Mix 2 tablespoons of any *cheese* into the potatoes and decrease the milk.
- Use *chicken broth* to boil the potatoes and use it instead of *milk.*
- Mix 2 tablespoons of *yogurt* or *sour cream.*

POTATO CROQUETTES

Prep time: 10 minutes
Cook time: 25 minutes

2 servings

Ingredients

2 medium potatoes, peeled and cut into slices
Water to cover the potatoes
1 medium egg beaten

1 teaspoon parsley
2 tablespoons flour
1/4 cup bread crumbs
2 tablespoons vegetable oil

Instructions

1. Put potatoes into the cold water to barely cover and bring to a boil.
2. Cook covered until potatoes are soft and can be poked easily with a fork and the water is absorbed.
3. Use a potato masher or a fork to mash the potatoes.
4. Add the egg, parsley, and flour so that the potato mixture is thick and can be molded into 4 patties.
5. Heat the oil in a fry pan.
6. Coat each patty in bread crumbs and fry it until brown. Turn once and fry the second side.
7. Put onto a paper towel to drain.

Nutrient Content

Calories 333
Protein 8 gm
9% calories from Protein
Carbohydrates 38 gm
Fat 17 gm

45% calories from Fat
Cholesterol 94 mg
Sodium 152 mg
Dietary Fiber 2 gm

Adaptations for Physical Limitations

- Adjust the consistency to the swallowing ability of the client by cutting the potatoes into small pieces.

Substitutions

- Add 1/4 cup grated **Parmesan cheese**.
- Vary spices used in the mashed potatoes.
- Serve with **applesauce** or **sour cream**.

ROSEMARY GARLIC SWEET POTATOES

Prep time: 5 minutes
Cook time: 30 minutes

4 servings

Ingredients

4 small sweet potatoes, washed and unpeeled (about 2 pounds)
2 tablespoons margarine

2 teaspoons dried rosemary
1 teaspoon garlic powder
Vegetable oil spray

Instructions

1. Preheat oven to 400°.
2. Cut each sweet potato into 6 wedges.
3. Melt margarine, rosemary, and garlic in saucepan.
4. Toss potato wedges in bowl with margarine mixture.
5. Place wedges on baking sheet. May spray with vegetable oil spray if desired.
6. Bake at 400° for 25–30 minutes or until tender.
7. Turn potatoes occasionally

Nutrient Content

Calories 190
Protein 2 gm
5% calories from Protein
Carbohydrates 32 gm
Fat 6 gm

28% calories from Fat
Cholesterol 0 mg
Sodium 84 mg
Dietary Fiber 4 gm

Adaptations for Physical Limitations

- Adjust the consistency to the swallowing ability of the client by cutting potatoes into small pieces.

Substitutions

- May sprinkle potatoes with ***brown sugar.***

ROASTED POTATOES

Prep time: 10 minutes
Cook time: 25 minutes

1 serving

Ingredients

1 medium potato cut into cubes, with or without the peel (wash the peel if left on)
Vegetable oil spray

$\frac{1}{4}$ teaspoon thyme, $\frac{1}{4}$ teaspoon rosemary, $\frac{1}{4}$ teapoon dill, and $\frac{1}{4}$ teaspoon parsley—mixed together

Instructions

1. Heat the oven to 350°.
2. Put the potatoes into a baking dish.
3. Spray the potatoes well with cooking oil spray and sprinkle with the herbs. Mix well.
4. Bake uncovered for about 25 minutes, turning once during cooking. Cook until the potatoes are soft.

Nutrient Content

Calories 100
Protein 3 gm
10% calories from Protein
Carbohydrates 22 gm
Fat 1 gm

10% calories from Fat
Cholesterol 0 mg
Sodium 8 mg
Dietary Fiber 2 gm

Adaptations for Physical Limitations

- Adjust the consistency to the swallowing ability of the client by cutting the potatoes into small pieces.

Substitutions

- Vary the spices used.
- Add some root vegetables such as *turnips, carrots, beets,* or *parsnips,* and roast together.

PASTA WITH BEANS

Prep time: 10 minutes
Cook time: 15 minutes

2 servings

Ingredients

6 ounces shell pasta, cooked and drained
Vegetable oil spray
$\frac{1}{2}$ cup chopped onion
$\frac{1}{2}$ cup chopped celery
$\frac{1}{2}$ cup grated carrot
1 clove minced garlic
3 leaves of Swiss chard or escarole, cut into small pieces

$\frac{1}{2}$ cup stewed tomatoes with juice
$\frac{1}{2}$ cup cannelloni beans, cooked and drained
$\frac{1}{2}$ cup green beans, cooked and drained
2 ounces grated Romano cheese

Instructions

1. Heat a large skillet sprayed with vegetable oil spray.
2. Cook the onions, celery, carrots, and garlic until soft.
3. Add the Swiss chard and cook for a few minutes until it wilts. (You may have to add a small bit of water to prevent sticking.)
4. Add the beans and tomatoes. Stir and cook about 2 minutes.
5. Add the pasta and heat thoroughly.
6. Sprinkle the cheese on top of the pasta as you serve it.

Nutrient Content

Calories 395
Protein 25 gm
25% calories from Protein
Carbohydrates 53 gm
Fat 10 gm

22% calories from Fat
Cholesterol 0 mg
Sodium 1022 mg
Dietary Fiber 8 gm

Adaptations for Physical Limitations

- Adjust the consistency to the swallowing ability of the client by cutting everything into small pieces, or pureeing in a blender. Add liquid to desired consistency.

Substitutions

- Vary the *beans.*
- Vary the *cheese* used.
- Add small *meat balls* or cut up cooked *chicken.*

PASTA WITH BUTTER

Prep time: 2 minutes
Cook time: 10 minutes

1 serving

Ingredients

2 ounces pasta, uncooked

2 teaspoons unsalted butter

Instructions

1. Fill a medium saucepan with water. Bring to a boil.
2. Put pasta into boiling water. Cover and bring back to a boil. Uncover.
3. Let boil until pasta is done to the preference of the client.
4. Drain. Do not rinse.
5. Put butter on it, mix, and serve.

Nutrient Content

Calories 280
Protein 7 gm
11% calories from Protein
Carbohydrates 43 gm
Fat 9 gm

28% calories from Fat
Cholesterol 21 mg
Sodium 5 mg
Dietary Fiber 1 gm

Adaptations for Physical Limitations

- Adjust the consistency to the swallowing ability of the client by cutting pasta into small pieces or pureeing in a blender. Add liquid to desired consistency.

Substitutions

- Sprinkle with 1–2 tablespoons of **cheese**.
- Sprinkle with $\frac{1}{4}$ teaspoon basil or oregano.
- Add $\frac{1}{2}$ cup cooked **vegetables** before serving.

PASTA WITH GARLIC AND OIL

Prep time: 2 minutes
Cook time: 10 minutes

2 servings

Ingredients

4 ounces pasta
2 tablespoons oil

2 cloves minced garlic

Instructions

1. Fill a medium saucepan with water. Bring to a boil.
2. Put pasta into boiling water. Cover and bring back to a boil. Uncover.
3. Let boil until pasta is done to the preference of the client.
4. Drain. Do not rinse.
5. Put olive oil and garlic on it and serve.

Nutrient Content

Calories 335
Protein 7 gm
9% calories from Protein
Carbohydrates 43 gm
Fat 15 gm

40% calories from Fat
Cholesterol 0 mg
Sodium 4 mg
Dietary Fiber 1 gm

Adaptations for Physical Limitations

- Adjust the consistency to the swallowing ability of the client by cutting the pasta into small pieces or pureeing in a blender. Add liquid to desired consistency.

Substitutions

- Add $\frac{1}{3}$ teaspoon basil or oregano.
- Add 1 teaspoon **grated cheese.**
- Add $\frac{1}{2}$ cup cooked **vegetables** before serving.

PASTA WITH HERBS AND CHEESE

Prep time: 4 minutes
Cook time: 10 minutes

2 servings

Ingredients

4 ounces pasta
6 ounces whole milk ricotta cheese
1 teaspoon oregano

1 tablespoon chives
1 clove garlic
2 tablespoons olive oil

Instructions

1. Fill a medium saucepan with water. Bring to a boil.
2. Put pasta into boiling water. Cover and bring back to a boil. Uncover.
3. Let boil until pasta is done to the preference of the client.
4. Drain. Do not rinse.
5. Meanwhile, mix the cheese, chives, oregano, and garlic together.
6. Combine the pasta, cheese, and olive oil.
7. Warm and serve.

Nutrient Content

Calories 486
Protein 17 gm
14% calories from Protein
Carbohydrates 48 gm
Fat 26 gm

48% calories from Fat
Cholesterol 41 mg
Sodium 77 mg
Dietary Fiber 2 gm

Adaptations for Physical Limitations

- Adjust the consistency to the swallowing ability of the client by cutting the pasta into small pieces or pureeing in a blender. Add liquid to desired consistency.

Substitutions

- Vary the **cheese** used to include small-curd cottage cheese, Parmesan, Jarlsberg, and cheddar.
- Add ½ cup cooked **vegetables** before serving.
- Add small **meatballs** or cup of cut up cooked **chicken**.

PASTA WITH QUICK TOMATO SAUCE

Prep time: 5 minutes
Cook time: 15 minutes

4 servings

Ingredients

8 ounces spaghetti, uncooked

1 recipe quick tomato sauce

Instructions

1. Fill a medium saucepan with water. Bring to a boil.
2. Put pasta into boiling water. Cover and bring back to a boil. Uncover.
3. Let boil until pasta is done to the preference of the client.
4. Drain. Do not rinse.
5. Heat Quick Tomato Sauce *(recipe located in Chapter 15)*
6. Combine sauce and spaghetti.

Nutrient Content

Calories 279
Protein 11 gm
16% calories from Protein
Carbohydrates 54 gm
Fat 1 gm

3% calories from Fat
Cholesterol 0mg
Sodium 7 mg
Dietary Fiber 2 gm

Adaptations for Physical Limitations

- Adjust the consistency to the swallowing ability of the client by cutting everything into very small pieces or pureeing in a blender. Add liquid to desired consistency.

Substitutions

- Sprinkle with **grated cheese**.
- Add hot pepper to taste.

BARLEY WITH MUSHROOMS

Prep time: 5 minutes
Cook time: 25 minutes

2 servings

Ingredients

Vegetable oil spray
¼ cup chopped onion
¼ cup chopped mushrooms

1 cup chicken broth
½ cup barley

Instructions

1. Spray sauce pan with vegetable oil spray and heat.
2. Cook the onions and mushrooms until light brown.
3. Add the barley and stir continuously until brown.
4. Add the chicken broth. Cover and cook until liquid is absorbed and barley is soft.

Nutrient Content

Calories 153
Protein 5 gm
13% calories from Protein
Carbohydrates 30 gm
Fat 2 gm

10% calories from Fat
Cholesterol 0 mg
Sodium 501 mg
Dietary Fiber 4 gm

Adaptations for Physical Limitations

- Adjust the consistency to the swallowing ability of the client by mashing the barley or pureeing in a blender. Add liquid to desired consistency.

Substitutions

- Use *vegetable broth* or *beef broth* to cook the barley.

GRITS CASSEROLE

Prep time: 5 minutes
Cook time: 75 minutes

6–8 servings

Ingredients

1 cup quick-cooking grits
4 cups boiling water
$\frac{1}{2}$ cup unsalted butter
1 medium egg, well beaten

5 ounces cheddar process cheese spread
1 tablespoon Worcestershire sauce
$\frac{1}{2}$ teaspoon hot pepper sauce
$\frac{1}{2}$ teaspoon garlic powder

Instructions

1. Preheat oven to 300°. In a large saucepan, slowly stir grits into boiling water.
2. Cook over medium heat for 5 minutes.
3. Stir in butter, egg, Worcestershire sauce, hot pepper sauce, and garlic powder.
4. Pour into shallow $1\frac{1}{2}$-quart casserole.
5. Bake for 60 to 75 minutes or until golden brown.

Nutrient Content

Calories 236
Protein 5 gm
9% calories from Protein
Carbohydrates 18 gm
Fat 16 gm

61% calories from Fat
Cholesterol 68 mg
Sodium 297 mg
Dietary Fiber 0 gm

Adaptations for Physical Limitations

- Adjust the consistency to the swallowing ability of the client by adding liquid if needed for thinner consistency.

Substitutions

- Add *salt* to taste.
- Add seasonings as desired.

QUINOA

Prep time: 4 minutes
Cook time: 25 minutes

2 servings

Ingredients

1 cup chicken broth

½ cup quinoa

Instructions

1. Bring chicken broth to a boil in a saucepan with cover.
2. Put quinoa into broth and simmer until all liquid is absorbed and grain is soft.

Nutrient Content

Calories 155
Protein 6 gm
16% calories from Protein
Carbohydrates 26 gm
Fat 3 gm

18% calories from Fat
Cholesterol 0 mg
Sodium 500 mg
Dietary Fiber 4 gm

Adaptations for Physical Limitations

- Adjust the consistency to the swallowing ability of the client by cooking grain thoroughly.

Substitutions

- Serve with **butter**.
- Vary **cooking liquid**.

TABBOULEH

Prep time: 25 minutes
Cook time: 0 minutes

4 servings

Ingredients

8 ounces bulgur wheat, uncooked
4 tablespoons green onion, chopped very small
1 cup tomato, chopped very small

4 cloves minced garlic
¼ cup lemon juice
4 tablespoons olive oil

Instructions

1. Put bulgur into a bowl and cover with cool water. Leave it there until the cereal is soft to the touch.
2. Line a colander with a clean kitchen towel. Drain the bulgur through the kitchen towel. Squeeze out all the water.
3. Put the dry bulgur into a bowl. Add all the other ingredients.
4. Mix well. Leave covered in refrigerator for at least 3 hours.

Nutrient Content

Calories 337
Protein 7 gm
8% calories from Protein
Carbohydrates 47 gm
Fat 16 gm

40% calories from Fat
Cholesterol 0 mg
Sodium 4 mg
Dietary Fiber 6 gm

Adaptations for Physical Limitations

- Adjust the consistency to the swallowing ability of the client by cutting everything into very small pieces.

Substitutions

- Vary the amount of lemon juice and *oil.*
- Add ¼ cup chopped mint.

CHAPTER 18

Recipes for Fruit

Introduction

Fruit provides minerals, vitamins, and fiber. Fruit can be eaten raw, cooked, alone, or as an ingredient in a simple or intricate dish. Fruit can add taste, texture, and color to any dish. Fruit is often served alone at the end of a meal or as a snack. It can, however, be an accompaniment to most any dish.

Before air travel, local fruits could be eaten only "in season." If a particular fruit was wanted for future use, it could be frozen or canned, but each variety of fresh fruit could be enjoyed for only a few months each year. With air travel and improved packing and storage techniques, almost all varieties of fruit can now be eaten year-round in most parts of the country. When choosing fruit, keep in mind the following:

- What appears freshest
- Choose fruit that is blemish free, plump, and has a good color
- Choose fruit that is ripe and ready to eat. If you must ripen fruit, leave it outside on a counter for a few days. Another method is to put fruit in a brown paper bag and leave it at room temperature until the fruit is ripened.
- Personal preference for ripeness should be respected. Some people like very ripe and soft fruit, and others like it less ripe and harder. Discuss this with your client.
- Choose fruit that will keep fresh. Most fruit will remain fresh in the refrigerator. It is best not to refrigerate bananas.

Peeling fruit is a matter of preference. Although some fruit, like citrus and bananas must be peeled before eating, other fruit like apples, peaches, etc. can be eaten either with or without the peel.

Always wash fruit before you serve it! It is wise to also wash fruit you will peel so that the bacteria from the peel does not transfer to the fruit as you peel it.

Recipes included in this chapter:

- Baked Apples
- Broiled Grapefruit
- Cooked Fruit Compote
- Fruit Cubes
- Glazed Bananas
- Nectarine and Cantaloupe Smoothie
- Pureed Fruit with Whipped Topping

Additional fruit recipes included in Chapter 22, Beverages:

- Blended Banana
- Fruit Freeze
- Strawberry Milk Smoothie
- Yogurt Smoothie

Additional fruit recipes included in Chapter 23, Snacks:

- Apple Crisp

BAKED APPLES

Prep time: 5 minutes
Cook time: 30 minutes

1 serving

Ingredients

1 McIntosh or Granny Smith apple
$\frac{1}{8}$ teaspoon cinnamon
1 teaspoon brown sugar, light or dark
$\frac{1}{4}$ teaspoon nutmeg

$\frac{1}{4}$ teaspoon unsalted butter
4 tablespoons water
5 raisins

Instructions

1. Preheat the oven to 350°.
2. Cut the top off the apple and core it.
3. Place the apple in a small baking dish.
4. Pack the hole of the apple with brown sugar and sprinkle nutmeg and cinnamon over the top.
5. Put the butter on the top of the apple.
6. Pour 4 tablespoons of water in the baking dish and put the raisins in the water.
7. Bake in the oven for about 30 minutes or until the apple is tender to a fork.

Nutrient Content

Calories 113
Protein 0 gm
1% calories from Protein
Carbohydrates 27 gm
Fat 2 gm

12% calories from Fat
Cholesterol 3 mg
Sodium 2 mg
Dietary Fiber 4 gm

Adaptations for Physical Limitations

- Adjust the consistency to the swallowing ability of the client by cutting the apple into small pieces or mashing it. You may have to remove the peel before serving.

Substitutions

- Use any type of apple.
- Use **margarine** in place of butter.
- Use **white sugar** instead of brown sugar.
- Use **apple juice** instead of water.
- Sprinkle $\frac{1}{8}$ teaspoon ground ginger over the apple.
- Season the apple after it has cooked with $\frac{1}{2}$ teaspoon lemon juice.

BROILED GRAPEFRUIT

Prep time: 5 minutes
Cook time: 10 minutes

2 servings

Ingredients

1 large grapefruit

2 tablespoons light brown sugar

Instructions

1. Cut grapefruit in half and remove seeds.
2. Cut around edge and sections to loosen grapefruit.
3. Remove center.
4. Sprinkle each half with 1 tablespoon brown sugar.
5. Broil grapefruit 6 inches away from heat for 5–10 minutes or until juice bubbles and edge turns lightly brown.
6. Serve hot.

Nutrient Content

Calories 89
Protein 1 gm
4% calories from Protein
Carbohydrates 23 gm
Fat 0 gm

2% calories from Fat
Cholesterol 0 mg
Sodium 4 mg
Dietary Fiber 2 gm

Adaptations for Physical Limitations

- Adjust the consistency to the swallowing ability of the client by cutting the grapefruit into small pieces. May not be appropriate for all clients

Substitutions

- Any variety of grapefruit can be used: white, pink, ruby red.
- Serve with **cottage cheese.**

COOKED FRUIT COMPOTE

Prep time: 10 minutes
Cook time: 25 minutes

3 servings

Ingredients

1 large apple cut into quarters, without pits

1 medium pear into quarters, without pits

1 cup nectarines in half, without the pit

2 apricots cut in half, without the pit

1 cup cherries cut in half, without the pit

1 cup water

1 tablespoon honey

Instructions

1. Put all ingredients into a saucepan and bring water to a boil.
2. Cook about 20 minutes or until fruit is soft but not mushy.
3. Allow to cool. May be served warm or cold.

Nutrient Content

Calories 156
Protein 2 gm
4% calories from Protein
Carbohydrates 39 gm
Fat 1 gm

6% calories from Fat
Cholesterol 0 mg
Sodium 3 mg
Dietary Fiber 5 gm

Adaptations for Physical Limitations

- Adjust the consistency to the swallowing ability of the client by cutting the fruit into small pieces or pureed. The fruit may have to be peeled before cooking.

Substitutions

- Any combination of fruit may be used.
- **Sugar** may be used instead of honey
- Season with any combination of lemon juice, cinnamon, or nutmeg.

FRUIT CUBES

Prep time: 5 minutes
Cook time: None

10 servings

Keep a supply in the freezer to add to any beverage.

Ingredients

4 nectarines, or peaches, washed and quartered, without pits

1 tablespoon lemon juice

Instructions

1. In a blender or food processor, blend fruit with lemon juice until smooth.
2. Pour into ice cube trays.
3. Freeze until firm.
4. Add to desired beverages.

Nutrient Content

Calories 27
Protein .5 gm
7% calories from Protein
Carbohydrates 7 gm
Fat 0 gm

7% calories from Fat
Cholesterol 0 mg
Sodium 0 mg
Dietary Fiber 1 gm

Adaptations for Physical Limitations

- None

Substitutions

- Remove skin from fruit before blending.
- Use any combination of fruits.

GLAZED BANANAS

Prep time: 5 minutes
Cook time: 7 minutes

2 servings

Ingredients

2 small bananas, peeled and cut in half lengthwise
1½ tablespoons unsalted butter

2 tablespoons brown sugar, light or dark
1 tablespoon lemon juice

Instructions

1. In a fry pan, heat the butter to melting point.
2. Put in the brown sugar and melt.
3. Put in the bananas.
4. Cook on one side for 2 minutes.
5. Turn and cook for another 2 minutes.
6. Put the lemon juice in. Coat the banana and remove to a plate.
7. Pour the syrup over the bananas and serve.

Nutrient Content

Calories 205
Protein 1 gm
2% calories from Protein
Carbohydrates 33 gm
Fat 9 gm

38% calories from Fat
Cholesterol 23 mg
Sodium 7 mg
Dietary Fiber 2 gm

Adaptations for Physical Limitations

- Adjust the consistency to the swallowing ability of the client by cutting the bananas into small pieces or mashing it with a fork.

Substitutions

- May be served with *yogurt* or *ice cream.*
- May be served with *whipped topping.*
- Serve over *pancakes.*

NECTARINE AND CANTALOUPE SMOOTHIE

Prep time: 10 minutes
Cook time: None

2 (1 1/4 cup) servings

Ingredients

1 nectarine, cut into cubes and skinned, without the pit
1 cup cantaloupe, diced, without skin
1/2 cup plain nonfat yogurt
1 teaspoon honey
3 ice cubes

Instructions

1. In blender, combine nectarine and cantaloupe.
2. Blend until smooth.
3. Add yogurt, honey, and ice. Blend until well blended.

Nutrient Content

Calories 105
Protein 5 gm
17% calories from Protein
Carbohydrates 22 gm
Fat 1 gm
5% calories from Fat
Cholesterol 1 mg
Sodium 55 mg
Dietary Fiber 2 gm

Adaptations for Physical Limitations

- Adjust the consistency to the swallowing ability of the client by blending longer if needed.

Substitutions

- *Low-fat yogurt* may be used.

PUREED FRUIT WITH WHIPPED TOPPING

Prep time: 15 minutes
Cook time: 20 minutes

2 servings

Ingredients

1 large apple cut into pieces
1 medium pear cut into pieces
1 cup cherries, pitted

1 cup water
1 cup whipped topping

Instructions

1. Put the fruit and water into a saucepan.
2. Boil until the fruit is soft and the liquid has boiled off.
3. Cool slightly and then force through a food mill or a sieve. Discard the skins.
4. Cool.
5. Mix with the whipped topping and serve.

Nutrient Content

Calories 254
Protein 1 gm
2% calories from Protein
Carbohydrates 46 gm
Fat 7 gm

26% calories from Fat
Cholesterol 0 mg
Sodium 4 mg
Dietary Fiber 6 gm

Adaptations for Physical Limitations

- None

Substitutions

- Any combination of fruit may be used.
- The **whipped topping** may be ***fat free*** or ***sugar free***.

CHAPTER 19

Recipes for Eggs and Cheese

Introduction

Eggs are very versatile food and are good sources of many of the nutrients needed for a healthy diet. Eggs contain protein and fat and many vitamins. Many diets, such as low-fat or low-cholesterol diets, limit the number of eggs. These limitations must be considered when planning meals since the eggs used in cooking are also counted in the weekly or daily number allowed. The yellow part of the eggs contain fat and cholesterol. The white part of the egg contains no fat only protein.

Eggs come in different colors, but they are all the same. The only difference is that different types of hens lay eggs of different colors. Some people prefer brown eggs; some people prefer white eggs. Respect that preference.

Eggs come in different sizes. You may use different sizes, but remember that the analysis will change slightly.

Egg substitutes are products that have removed the fat and cholesterol. They are available in the frozen food section and the egg section of most supermarkets. They cannot always be used interchangeably with fresh eggs. They can, however, be used in these recipes. There may be a slight difference in the finished food, but if there is serious consideration as to the amount of fat and/or cholesterol, this option should be considered. If there is more than one egg in the recipe, egg substitute may be used for one of the eggs. Egg whites can also be substituted for up to half of the egg requirement in the recipe.

Eggs in their shell should always be refrigerated. **<u>Never use an egg that is cracked</u>**. Eggs that are cracked can cause food-borne illnesses.

Cheese is a useful and versatile food. It does, however, contain a large proportion of fat. Its use should be balanced throughout the day and week. All cheese, whether it is eaten plain or used in cooking, must be taken into consideration when reviewing the dietary intake of your client. Some cheeses are available in low-sodium and/or low-fat varieties. Although these cheeses retain their basic taste, they do taste somewhat different. They also respond to cooking slightly differently than their more fatty versions. Discuss with your client which version is preferred and take that as well as the client's dietary restriction into consideration when planning all the meals.

All recipes are presented using whole milk and whole medium eggs. The cheese is also regular cheese unless low fat is indicated. If the client has a reduced-fat, -cholesterol, -sodium and/or -calorie diet, the products that are low fat and low sodium should be substituted. Using the low-fat and low-sodium varieties will change the nutrient content of the recipe. Refer to Table C in the Appendix for specific nutrient content.

Recipes included in this chapter:

- Blintzes
- Cheese Filling for Blintzes
- Cheese Quesadillas
- Egg Salad
- French Toast
- Frittata
- Omelet
- Quiche
- Strata

BLINTZES

Prep time: 35 minutes
Cook time: 25 minutes

4 (2 blintzes) servings

Ingredients

2/3 cup all-purpose flour
1 cup milk

3 eggs
Vegetable oil spray

Note: Blintzes, also know as crepes, may be stuffed with cheese, jelly, fruit, or meat. They should always be reheated in an oven or skillet before eating.

Instructions

1. Mix the flour, milk, and eggs in a pitcher or bowl. Cover it and refrigerate for at least 30 minutes or up to 1 day.
2. Spray a crepe pan or small skillet with vegetable spray and heat.
3. Pour 2–3 tablespoons of batter into middle of pan and tilt the pan so that the entire bottom surface is covered.
4. Cook this side until it is light brown and the crepe appears dry, about 2–3 minutes.
5. Lift a corner of the crepe to check
6. Turn the crepe over and cook another 30 seconds.
7. Remove the crepe to a plate and cover with wax paper so next crepe can be placed on top of the paper.
8. When you are finished, wrap the stack in tin foil and save until ready to be stuffed. They may be frozen at this point.

Nutrient Content

Calories 170
Protein 9 gm
22% calories from Protein
Carbohydrates 20 gm
Fat 5 gm

29% calories from Fat
Cholesterol 143 mg
Sodium 74 mg
Dietary Fiber 0 gm

Adaptations for Physical Limitations

- Adjust the consistency to the swallowing ability of the client by cutting into appropriate size pieces.

Substitutions

- Any flavored flour may be used with white flour such as chestnut, almond, buckwheat, rye, whole wheat. The liquid may have to be adjusted.
- Any *milk* may be used including fat free evaporated or condensed.
- *Egg substitutes* may be used.

CHEESE FILLING FOR BLINTZES

Prep time: 5 minutes
Cook time: 3 minutes

4 servings

Ingredients

1 cup 2% cottage cheese
½ cup vanilla yogurt

1 teaspoon sugar

Instructions

1. Drain the cottage cheese if there is a lot of liquid.
2. Combine all ingredients. Mix well.
3. Keep covered and refrigerated until ready to use in the blintzes.
4. When ready to fill blintzes:
   a. Put about 3-4 tablespoons of filling in the middle of a blintz.
   b. Fold the edges over the filling and put it into a warm pan with the folded edges down.
   c. Slide the warmed blintz onto a plate.
   d. Garnish with jelly, sour cream, yogurt, or sugar.

Nutrient Content

Calories 65
Protein 8 gm
53% calories from Protein
Carbohydrates 5 gm
Fat 1 gm

15% calories from Fat
Cholesterol 0
Sodium 248 mg
Dietary Fiber 0 gm

Adaptations for Physical Limitations

- Adjust the consistency to the swallowing ability of the client by cutting the blintzes into small pieces.

Substitutions

- Any flavor **yogurt** may be used.
- Tablespoon of any flavor **jelly** may be added.
- **Yogurt** may be replaced with **sour cream.**
- **Yogurt** may be omitted.
- Any type or flavor of **cottage cheese** may be used.

CHEESE QUESADILLAS

Prep time: 15 minutes
Cook time: 10 minutes

2 servings

Ingredients

4 flour tortillas
3 ounces sharp cheddar cheese, grated
3 tablespoons chopped red onion

4 tablespoons salsa
Vegetable oil spray

Instructions

1. Lay two tortillas on counter.
2. Spread half the salsa on each one.
3. Sprinkle half the cheese and half the onion on each one.
4. Cover it with the other tortilla.
5. Spray a skillet with vegetable spray and heat.
6. Gently place one quesadilla in the pan and cook until the cheese melts and the tortilla is brown. If needed, spray the top tortilla with vegetable spray and turn the quesadilla to cook the second side.
7. Put on a plate and cut into quarters.
8. Serve immediately.

Nutrient Content

Calories 554
Protein 22 gm
16% calories from Protein
Carbohydrates 72 gm
Fat 20 gm

32% calories from Fat
Cholesterol 30 mg
Sodium 1088 mg
Dietary Fiber .6 gm

Adaptations for Physical Limitations

- Adjust the consistency to the swallowing ability of the client by cutting the quesadilla into appropriate size pieces.

Substitutions

- Any type of *cheese* may be used.
- Any type of tortilla may be used.
- Any type of spice and/or vegetable may be used such as broccoli, green pepper, celery, zucchini, tomatoes, lettuce.
- *Sour cream* or *yogurt* may be spread in the quesadilla before cooking.
- Hot spice or hot peppers may be added before cooking.

EGG SALAD

Prep time: 2 minutes
Cook time: 10 minutes

1 serving

Ingredients

1 egg, hard-boiled and shelled
1 tablespoon mayonnaise

2 tablespoons diced celery

Instructions

1. Mix all ingredients.
2. Serve with bread, crackers, or vegetables.
3. Either refrigerate or eat immediately.

Nutrient Content

Calories 167
Protein 6 gm
14% calories from Protein
Carbohydrates 1 gm
Fat 15 gm

84% calories from Fat
Cholesterol 197 mg
Sodium 143 mg
Dietary Fiber 0 gm

Adaptations for Physical Limitations

- Adjust the consistency to the swallowing ability of the client by either mashing the egg or adding additional *mayonnaise*.

Substitutions

- Any type of *mayonnaise* may be used.
- Vary spices, including dill, mustard, thyme, or garlic.
- Add lemon juice.
- Add *carrots,* finely diced *onions,* or green or red *peppers* to egg mixture.

FRENCH TOAST

Prep time: 5 minutes
Cook time: 8 minutes

2 servings

Ingredients

2 medium eggs
4 slices white bread, slightly soft

Vegetable oil spray

Instructions

1. Break the eggs into a flat plate with sides. Beat them until well blended.
2. Spray a frying pan with the vegetable oil spray.
3. Heat the pan on medium heat.
4. Dip each piece of bread into egg. Allow the bread to stay in the egg for a few minutes to absorb the egg.
5. Carefully transfer bread to frying pan.
6. Fry the bread to a golden brown on both sides. If the bread sticks to the pan, spray the pan again.
7. Serve hot.

Nutrient Content

Calories 206
Protein 9.5 gm
18% calories from Protein
Carbohydrates 29 gm
Fat 6 gm

27% calories from Fat
Cholesterol 187 mg
Sodium 325 mg
Dietary Fiber 0 gm

Adaptations for Physical Limitations

- Adjust the size of cut bread to the client's ability to swallow. If necessary can be pureed in blender by adding small amount of liquid such as milk.

Substitutions

- May be served with any type of **syrup, sugar,** and/or **butter.**
- Add 1 tablespoon of cinnamon to the egg before dipping the bread.
- Any type of bread may be used.
- May be cooked in **butter.**

FRITTATA

Prep time: 10 minutes
Cook time: 10 minutes

1 serving

Ingredients

1 medium egg
1 tablespoon chopped tomato
1 tablespoon chopped onion
1 ounce grated cheddar cheese
1 tablespoon grated Parmesan cheese
½ teaspoon dried basil
Vegetable oil spray

Instructions

1. Beat the egg with the basil.
2. Spray a skillet with vegetable spray and heat it.
3. Pour the egg into the skillet.
4. Add the tomato, onion, cheddar cheese, and Parmesan. Do not mix.
5. Continue to cook until the egg is cooked and firm.
6. Loosen the sides and slide the frittata onto a plate.

Nutrient Content

Calories 186
Protein 15 gm
34% calories from Protein
Carbohydrates 3 gm
Fat 12 gm
60% calories from Fat
Cholesterol 211 mg
Sodium 390 mg
Dietary Fiber .5 gm

Adaptations for Physical Limitations

- Adjust the size of each bite to the client's ability to swallow. If necessary, the egg can be mashed.

Substitutions

- Any type of **cheese** or combination of cheese may be used.
- Any type or combination of **vegetable** may be used.
- Vary the spices.

OMELET

Prep time: 2 minutes
Cook time: 4 minutes

1 serving

Ingredients

1 medium egg

Vegetable oil spray

Instructions

1. Beat the egg until well blended.
2. Spray the frying pan with vegetable oil spray.
3. Heat the frying pan over medium heat.
4. Pour the egg into the pan and roll the pan so that the entire bottom is covered with egg.
5. Let the egg cook until it is set. Check the bottom of the egg by slipping a fork or thin spatula until the edge of the egg and lifting gently.
6. When the bottom is set, using a small spatula, gently lift half the egg and fold it over the other half. Let it cook another 30 seconds.
7. Slip the whole egg onto a plate and serve.

Nutrient Content

Calories 66
Protein 6 gm
34% calories from Protein
Carbohydrates .5 gm
Fat 4 grams

62% calories from Fat
Cholesterol 187 mg
Sodium 55 mg
Dietary Fiber 0 gm

Adaptations for Physical Limitations

- Adjust the size each piece of egg to the client's ability to swallow. If necessary the egg can be mashed.

Substitutions

- Any type of **cheese,** 1–2 tablespoons per egg, can be added to the omelet before it is finished cooking.
- Any type of **vegetable,** can be added to the omelet before it is finished cooking. Vegetables should be raw if they are quick cooking or precooked if they usually require a long cooking time.
- Vary spices used.

QUICHE

Prep time: 15 minutes
Cook time: 45 minutes

6 servings

Ingredients

1 9-inch pie shell
4 medium eggs
2 cups half and half

12 ounces grated Swiss cheese
8 ounces grated Parmesan cheese
½ cup chopped onion

Instructions

1. Preheat the oven to 350°.
2. Bake the pie shell for 5 minutes.
3. Mix the eggs, cheese, and onions well.
4. Pour the liquid into the pie shell.
5. Bake until the pie is set and a knife inserted into the center comes out clean. About 40 minutes.
6. Cool 10 minutes and serve.

Nutrient Content

Calories 667
Protein 40 gm
24% calories from Protein
Carbohydrates 19 gm
Fat 48 grams

65% calories from Fat
Cholesterol 234 mg
Sodium 952 mg
Dietary Fiber 0 gm

Adaptations for Physical Limitations

- Adjust the size of the pieces to the ability of the client to swallow. May be mashed.

Substitutions

- Any type of **hard cheese** may be used. Amount of total cheese may vary up to ¼ cup. Some **low-fat cheese** may be used.
- **Milk, cream,** and **half and half** may be used in any combination. If only milk is used, add an egg. Some **fat-free or skim milk** may be used. **Condensed skim milk** may be used.
- Vary spices.
- Eliminate onions if desired.
- Cooked **crabmeat, fish,** or **seafood** may be added (up to ¾ cup).
- Add ½ cup cooked **sausage**.

STRATA

Prep time: 15 minutes
Refrigerate overnight

Cook time: 40 minutes
4 servings

Ingredients

4 slices day-old white bread
3 medium eggs
¼ cup milk
4 ounces sharp cheddar cheese, grated
½ cup broccoli

2 ounces chopped cooked ham
¼ cup chopped raw onion
¾ teaspoon garlic powder
1 tablespoon dried parsley
Vegetable oil spray

Instructions

1. Spray a baking dish with vegetable oil spray that will hold the bread in two layers.
2. Mix the egg, milk, garlic powder, parsley, and rosemary together.
3. Place one layer of bread in the pan. Sprinkle half of the ham, broccoli, and cheese over the bread.
4. Place another layer of bread and sprinkle the remaining ham, broccoli, and cheese over the bread.
5. Pour the egg mixture over the bread. Allow the bread to absorb some of the egg mixture. Cover and refrigerate overnight.
6. When ready to cook, preheat the oven to 350°.
7. Place the strata uncovered in the oven and bake until the cheese is brown, about 40 minutes.
8. Let sit for 5 minutes before cutting.

Nutrient Content

Calories 229
Protein 17 gm
30% calories from Protein
Carbohydrates 14 gm
Fat 10 grams

43% calories from Fat
Cholesterol 289 mg
Sodium 540 mg
Dietary Fiber 1 gm

Adaptations for Physical Limitations

- Adjust the size of cut bread to the client's ability to swallow. May be mashed.

Substitutions

- Any type of at least day old bread can be used. The absorption of the egg mixture will vary with different breads.
- Any type of *cheese* or combination of cheese may be used.
- Any type of cooked or partially cooked meat or combination of meat can be used. **Do not use partially cooked chicken. Chicken must be completely cooked before using.**
- Any type of *vegetables* or combination of *vegetable* can be used.
- Vary spices.
- May be frozen after it is cooked.

CHAPTER 20

Recipes for Salad

Introduction

Salads are very versatile and add a great deal of variety to the meal. Salad may be served before the main course, after the main course, or with the main course. Ask the client when he or she is used to eating salad. If a salad has the protein for the meal in it, it can be served as the main course.

Salads provide fiber, bulk, and many vitamins not found in other foods.

Making a salad is an individual affair. Each person does it slightly differently.

- Some people wash their lettuce before they store it in the refrigerator. Some wash it right before they use it.
- Some people cut their lettuce. Some people tear it.
- Some people cut their tomatoes and other vegetables in chunks, some cut them in circles.
- Some people put the salad dressing directly on the salad and toss it before they bring it to the table and some people bring the salad dressing to the table in a small pitcher and pour it on each serving.
- Some people serve salad on different plates from the ones used for the main course.

Each person enjoys a different amount of salad dressing. The measurements in the recipes are a guide. You should discuss with your client his or her individual preferences for:

- Amount of salad dressing
- Tartness or sweetness
- Use of salt and pepper
- Use of low-fat and low-salt products

It is always important to keep the salad fresh. If the dressing contains mayonnaise, the dish should always be kept in the refrigerator until ready to be served and then kept out only as long as necessary.

Salad ingredients should be kept individually wrapped in dish towels or plastic bags in the drawers of the refrigerator.

Recipes included in this chapter:

- Carrot and Raisin Salad
- Chef's Salad
- Cole Slaw
- Potato Salad
- Rice and Vegetable Salad
- Spinach Salad
- Three-Bean Salad
- Tuna Fish Salad
- Vegetable Salad

Recipes for salad dressings:

- Balsamic Vinaigrette
- Basic Lemon Dressing
- Blue Cheese Dressing
- Lemon Garlic Mayonnaise

CARROT AND RAISIN SALAD

Prep time: 10 minutes
Cook time: None

4 servings

Ingredients

2½ cups peeled, shredded carrots
⅓ cup raisins
1 teaspoon lemon juice

¼ cup sour cream
¼ cup mayonnaise

Instructions

1. Combine the carrots and the raisins in a large bowl.
2. Combine the lemon juice, sour cream and mayonnaise and mix well.
3. Pour the dressing over the carrots and mix well.
4. Refrigerate until ready to serve.

Nutrient Content

Calories 197
Protein 2 gm
3% calories from Protein
Carbohydrates 17 gm
Fat 14 gm

63% calories from Fat
Cholesterol 16 mg
Sodium 108 mg
Dietary Fiber 3 gm

Adaptations for Physical Limitations

- Adjust the consistency to the swallowing ability of the client by shredding the carrots well. May have to cut the raisins into small pieces. Puree in blender if needed.

Substitutions

- Any type of *mayonnaise* may be used.
- Substitute plain *yogurt* for the sour cream.
- Omit the lemon juice.
- Omit the *raisins*.
- Add ½ cup *apple* cut into small pieces.

CHEF'S SALAD

Prep time: 15 minutes
Cook time: None

4 servings

Ingredients

5 cups chopped lettuce
1 medium chopped tomato
8 ounces cooked turkey, cut into long strips

4 ounces American cheese, cut into strips
4 ounces ham, cut into strips
1 large hard-boiled egg, quartered

Note: two servings dressing of choice is not included in the analysis.

Instructions

1. Arrange the lettuce in a bowl.
2. Lay the tomato, turkey, cheese, ham, and egg over the lettuce.
3. Dress the salad with dressing of choice.

Nutrient Content

Calories 248
Protein 27 gm
44% calories from Protein
Carbohydrates 6 gm
Fat 13 gm

46% calories from Fat
Cholesterol 93 mg
Sodium 798 mg
Dietary Fiber 1.3 gm

Adaptations for Physical Limitations

- Adjust the consistency to the swallowing ability of the client by cutting the salad into small pieces. May not be appropriate for all clients.

Substitutions

- Vary the *cheese* used, including low-fat varieties.
- Omit the *egg*.
- Add other vegetables such as ½ cup sliced *carrots*, ½ cup sliced *celery*, ¼ cup sliced *onion*.
- Vary salad dressing, including **low-fat varieties**.
- Use **cooked sliced beef**.
- Cooked *vegetables* may be added.

COLE SLAW

Prep time: 15 minutes
Cook time: None

4 servings

Ingredients

2 cups shredded raw cabbage (green, red, or mixed)
¼ cup shredded raw peeled carrot
¼ cup mayonnaise
1 tablespoon white distilled vinegar
½ teaspoon sugar

Instructions

1. Mix the cabbage and the carrot in a large bowl.
2. Mix the mayonnaise, vinegar, and sugar.
3. Pour the mayonnaise mixture over the cabbage and mix well.
4. Keep covered and refrigerated until ready to eat

Nutrient Content

Calories 114
Protein .6 gm
2% calories from Protein
Carbohydrates 3 gm
Fat 11 gm

87% calories from Fat
Cholesterol 10 mg
Sodium 89 mg
Dietary Fiber 1 gm

Adaptations for Physical Limitations

- Adjust the consistency to the swallowing ability of the client by cutting the cabbage into small pieces. May not be appropriate for all clients.

Substitutions

- Any type of *mayonnaise* may be used.
- Wine vinegar may be used instead of white vinegar.
- Substitute *sour cream* for some of the *mayonnaise.*

POTATO SALAD

Prep time: 15 minutes
Cook time: None

Refrigeration time: 1 hour
2 servings

Ingredients

2 cups boiled sliced potatoes, with or without the skin
½ cup sliced celery
¼ cup sliced onion

½ cup shredded carrots
3 tablespoons mayonnaise
1 teaspoon dill

Instructions

1. Combine all ingredients in a large bowl.
2. Cover and refrigerate at least 1 hour before serving.

Nutrient Content

Calories 158
Protein 2 gm
5% calories from Protein
Carbohydrates 19 gm
Fat 8 gm

48% calories from Fat
Cholesterol 7.5 mg
Sodium 82 mg
Dietary Fiber 3 gm

Adaptations for Physical Limitations

- Adjust the consistency to the swallowing ability of the client by cutting all ingredient into small pieces.

Substitutions

- Add 1 teaspoon prepared mustard.
- Add 1 teaspoon lemon juice.
- Add ¼ cup diced **green and/or red pepper.**
- Add 1 mashed hard-boiled **egg.**
- Vary the dressing including **vinaigrette.**
- Add cooked **vegetables.**

RICE AND VEGETABLE SALAD

Prep time: 10 minutes
Cook time: None

4 servings

Ingredients

3 cups cooked, cooled rice
1/3 cup chopped red pepper
1/3 cup chopped green pepper
1/2 cup sliced onion
1/2 cup raisins

1/2 cup broccoli flowerets
1/2 cup thawed frozen peas
1/4 cup fresh parsley
4 tablespoons red wine vinegar
1 tablespoon vegetable oil

Instructions

1. Combine all ingredients except the dressing in a large bowl.
2. Pour the dressing on when ready to serve.

Nutrient Content

Calories 273
Protein 5 gm
8% calories from Protein
Carbohydrates 54 gm
Fat 4 gm

13% calories from Fat
Cholesterol 0 mg
Sodium 481 mg
Dietary Fiber 3 gm

Adaptations for Physical Limitations

- Adjust the consistency to the swallowing ability of the client by cutting all the ingredients into small pieces.

Substitutions

- Vary the *vegetables* used.
- Omit the *raisins*.
- Use *vinaigrette* dressing in place of vinegar and oil.
- Vary the *salad dressing*.
- Add 1/4 cup *nuts*.
- Add 1/4 cup *cheese*.

SPINACH SALAD

Prep time: 10 minutes
Cook time: None

4 servings

Ingredients

4 cups raw spinach, very well washed
4 tablespoons olive oil
2 tablespoons apple cider vinegar
1 teaspoon sugar
2 ounces feta cheese crumbled
1 large hard-boiled egg, shelled

Instructions

1. Tear the spinach into a bowl.
2. Mix the olive oil, vinegar, and sugar well in a container.
3. Pour the salad dressing over the spinach.
4. Crumble the cheese and the egg over the spinach.

Nutrient Content

Calories 232
Protein 10 gm
16% calories from Protein
Carbohydrates 10 gm
Fat 19 gm

68% calories from Fat
Cholesterol 66 mg
Sodium 654 mg
Dietary Fiber 4 gm

Adaptations for Physical Limitations

- Adjust the consistency to the swallowing ability of the client by cutting the spinach into small pieces.

Substitutions

- Vary the vinegar, the *oil,* and the *cheese.*
- Omit the *egg.*
- Top with crumbled *bacon.*

THREE-BEAN SALAD

Prep time: 10 minutes
Cook time: None

Refrigeration time: 1 hour
4 servings

Ingredients

1 cup sliced red onion
½ cup black beans, cooked, cooled, and washed
½ cup green beans, cooked and cooled
½ cup garbanzo beans, cooked, cooled, and washed

¼ cup olive oil
2 tablespoons balsamic vinegar
½ teaspoon garlic powder

Instructions

1. Combine the onions and the beans in a large bowl.
2. Combine the olive oil, vinegar, and garlic powder in a bowl. Mix well.
3. Combine the dressing with the beans.
4. Refrigerate at least 1 hour before serving.

Nutrient Content

Calories 190
Protein 4 gm
8% calories from Protein
Carbohydrates 15 gm
Fat 15 gm

64% calories from Fat
Cholesterol 0 mg
Sodium 161 mg
Dietary Fiber 2 gm

Adaptations for Physical Limitations

- Adjust the consistency to the swallowing ability of the client by cutting the beans and onions into small pieces. May be mashed.

Substitutions

- Vary the vinegar.
- Combine any cooked, canned **beans.** Be sure to wash them well before using them.

TUNA FISH SALAD

Prep time: 10 minutes
Cook time: None

1 serving

Ingredients

3 ounces white albacore tuna packed in water, drained
¼ cup chopped celery

1 tablespoon mayonnaise

Instructions

1. Combine all ingredients.
2. Keep refrigerated until ready to eat.

Nutrient Content

Calories 195
Protein 21 gm
41% calories from Protein
Carbohydrates 3 gm
Fat 13 gm

54% calories from Fat
Cholesterol 5 mg
Sodium 471 mg
Dietary Fiber .5 gm

Adaptations for Physical Limitations

- Adjust the consistency to the swallowing ability of the client by mashing the ingredients well.

Substitutions

- Add 2 tablespoons of chopped *onion, carrots,* or *green onions.*
- Use any variety of *mayonnaise.*

VEGETABLE SALAD

Prep time: 10 minutes
Cook time: None

Refrigeration time: 30 minutes
2 servings

Ingredients

½ cup cooked broccoli, cut into small pieces
½ cup cooked carrots, cup into small pieces
½ cup cooked green beans, cut into small pieces
½ cup cooked cauliflower, cut into small pieces
2 tablespoons Italian salad dressing

Instructions

1. Combine all ingredients in bowl.
2. Chill for at least 30 minutes before serving.

Nutrient Content

Calories 113
Protein 3 gm
9% calories from Protein
Carbohydrates 11 gm
Fat 7.5 gm
55 % calories from Fat
Cholesterol 0 mg
Sodium 165 mg
Dietary Fiber 4 gm

Adaptations for Physical Limitations

- Adjust the consistency to the swallowing ability of the client by cutting the vegetables into small pieces. May be pureed. Add liquid to desired consistency.

Substitutions

- Vary the vegetables—*peas, brussels sprouts, zucchini* are excellent.
- Vary the *salad dressing.*
- Add 2 tablespoons *grated cheese.*
- Add ½ teaspoon of prepared mustard.

BALSAMIC VINAIGRETTE

Prep time: 5 minutes
Cook time: None

4 servings

Ingredients

4 tablespoons olive oil
2 tablespoons balsamic vinegar

$\frac{1}{2}$ teaspoon salt
$\frac{1}{4}$ teaspoon pepper

Instructions

1. Thoroughly mix all ingredients.

Nutrient Content

Calories 131
Protein 0 gm
0% from Protein
Carbohydrates 2 gm
Fat 14 gm

93% calories from Fat
Cholesterol 0 mg
Sodium 176 mg
Dietary Fiber 0 gm

Substitutions

- Vary the type of vinegar to include any flavored vinegar.
- Vary seasoning to include dill, thyme, rosemary, and tarragon.
- Vary type of oil to include any flavored oil except peanut.
- Add $\frac{1}{2}$ teaspoon of prepared mustard.

BASIC LEMON DRESSING

Prep time: 5 minutes
Cook time: None

4 servings

Ingredients

4 tablespoons olive oil
2 tablespoons lemon juice

$\frac{1}{2}$ teaspoon garlic powder
$\frac{1}{4}$ teaspoon pepper

Instructions

1. Thoroughly mix all ingredients in a bowl or jar.
2. Adjust seasoning to taste.

Nutrient Content

Calories 123
Protein 0 gm
0% calories from Protein
Carbohydrates 1 gm
Fat 14 gm

97% calories from Fat
Cholesterol 0 mg
Sodium 3 mg
Dietary Fiber 0 gm

Substitutions

- Vary the type of acid to include any *citrus juice.*
- Vary seasoning to include, salt, thyme, rosemary.

BLUE CHEESE DRESSING

Prep time: 5 minutes
Cook time: None

6 servings

Ingredients

1 cup mayonnaise
1 cup buttermilk
½ teaspoon garlic powder

1 tablespoon Worcestershire sauce
8 ounces crumbled blue cheese, divided
1 tablespoon sour cream

Instructions

1. Combine half of the blue cheese with all the other ingredients.
2. Mix well. May use blender at low speed.
3. Add remaining blue cheese and mix.
4. Serve.
5. Store in refrigerator.

Nutrient Content

Calories 292
Protein 2 gm
2% calories from Protein
Carbohydrates 2 gm
Fat 30 gm

94% calories from Fat
Cholesterol 15 mg
Sodium 305 mg
Dietary Fiber 0 gm

Adaptations for Physical Limitations

- Blend all ingredients until desired consistency.

Substitutions

- Use any **imitation mayonnaise** or variety of **mayonnaise**.
- Serve over **hamburger** or **broiled chicken**.

LEMON GARLIC MAYONNAISE

Prep time: 5 minutes
Cook time: None

4 servings

Ingredients

1 tablespoon lemon juice
½ cup mayonnaise

1½ teaspoons garlic powder

Instructions

1. Mix all ingredients thoroughly.

Nutrient Content

Calories 204
Protein 0 gm
0% calories from Protein
Carbohydrates 1 gm
Fat 22 gm

98% calories from Fat
Cholesterol 10 mg
Sodium 161 mg
Dietary Fiber 0 gm

Adaptations for Physical Limitations

- None

Substitutions

- Add ¼ teaspoon garlic powder.
- Add ¼ teaspoon dill.

CHAPTER 21

Recipes for Sandwiches

Introduction

Sandwiches are a very useful part of a total nutrition plan. They provide:

- A means to vary the way the client eats
- A way to use leftovers
- A way to prepare snacks and meals quickly
- A way to prepare a nourishing meal in advance
- A great way to vary diet and increase choices of food

Sandwiches are foods that are served between two pieces of bread. They can also be food that is served with a tortilla wrapped around it or a food that is slipped in the pocket of pita bread.

They may be served as a main course, as a snack, or as part of a meal. Anything you can put between two slices of bread or on a roll is a good sandwich. Use your imagination!

A sandwich has several parts, all of which are variable:

- *The bread:* White, rye, whole wheat, Italian, French, pita, tortilla, Portuguese, sourdough, pumpernickel, toasted.
- *The spread (what you put on the bread):* mustard, mayonnaise, ketchup, oil, vinegar
- *The major filling or contents (what you put in the sandwich, such as vegetables, meat, fish, salad):* A slice of filling in the recipes to follow generally refers to one ounce.
- *The accompaniments:* pickles, lettuce, tomatoes, onions, hot peppers, cheese, yogurt, horseradish, hoisin sauce, pesto, tomato sauce
- *The manner in which the sandwich is cut:* in half, thirds, quarters, or left whole you are encouraged to experiment and change the variables as your client will tolerate.

It is important that you discuss with your client the elements he likes to remain the same and the elements that can change. For instance, a client may always like his sandwiches on white bread with mayonnaise regardless of what the major component of the sandwich is. Some clients like salad dressing and not mayonnaise.

Following is a list of breads, fillings, and accompaniments. The combinations are endless. Find out what your clients like to eat and create your own recipe.

Ideas for Filling or Contents
Assorted cold cuts
Bacon
Canned luncheon meats
Cheese
Chicken salad
Egg salad
Jelly
Peanut butter
Sliced cooked beef
Sliced cooked chicken
Sliced cooked ham
Sliced cooked lamb
Sliced cooked pork
Sliced cooked roast beef
Sliced cooked turkey
Sliced hard-cooked eggs
Softened cream cheese
Tuna salad

Ideas for Bread
Biscuits
Corn muffins
English muffin
Frankfurter bun
Hamburger bun
Hoagie roll
Kaiser roll
Onion bread or roll
Pita bread
Potato bread or roll
Pumpernickel bread
Raisin bread
Rye bread
Tortilla wrap
Vienna bread
White bread
Whole-wheat bread

Ideas for the Accompaniments
Fresh spinach
Lettuce, all kinds
Sliced cucumbers
Sliced green or red peppers
Sliced onions
Sliced radishes
Spanish olives

Safety issues associated with eating sandwich are:

- Be sure the client can bite and chew all the contents of the sandwich.
- Be sure the client is not surprised by one of the contents, like a hot pepper he may not have expected.
- Be sure the client can hold the sandwich comfortably and has the ability to take small bites of it.
- Be sure the client can control the sandwich and that part of it will not slip out and soil his clothes, create a mess, or waste the food.
- Be sure the contents remain fresh until the sandwich is eaten.

Recipes included in this chapter:

- English Muffin Pizza
- Grilled Cheese
- Roasted Vegetable Sandwich
- Turkey and Cheese Roll-up

ENGLISH MUFFIN PIZZA

Prep time: 5 minutes
Cook time: 3 minutes

1 serving

Ingredients

1 English muffin
¼ teaspoon oregano
¼ teaspoon basil

2 teaspoons Italian tomato sauce
1 ounce mozzarella cheese

Instructions

1. Toast the muffin until light brown.
2. Spread the tomato sauce over the toasted inside of the muffin.
3. Sprinkle the dried herbs on the muffin.
4. Put the cheese over the tomato sauce.
5. Place in the microwave for 30 seconds or under the broiler until the cheese is bubbly.

Nutrient Content

Calories 220
Protein 12 gm
22% calories from Protein
Carbohydrates 29 gm
Fat 6 gm

24% calories from Fat
Cholesterol 16 mg
Sodium 387 mg
Dietary Fiber 0 gm

Adaptations for Physical Limitations

- Adjust the consistency to the swallowing ability of the client by cutting the muffin into small pieces.

Substitutions

- Add a few slices of mushrooms, **pepperoni,** or **sausage** under the cheese.
- Use a **bagel** instead of an English muffin.

GRILLED CHEESE

Prep time: 3 minutes
Cook time: 6 minutes

1 serving

Ingredients

2 slices white bread
2 ounces American cheese (yellow or white)

Vegetable oil spray

Instructions

1. Spray a frying pan well with the vegetable oil spray. Heat.
2. Put the cheese between two pieces of bread and place in the frying pan.
3. When one side is brown, turn and fry the other side. You may have to add more spray.

Nutrient Content

Calories 350
Protein 16 gm
18% calories from Protein
Carbohydrates 26 gm
Fat 20 gm

52% calories from Fat
Cholesterol 0 mg
Sodium 1140 mg
Dietary Fiber 0 gm

Adaptations for Physical Limitations

- Adjust the consistency to the swallowing ability of the client by cutting the sandwich into small pieces.

Substitutions

- Use any type of **hard cheese,** like **Swiss** or **cheddar.**
- Add **meat** and/or tomato between the slices of cheese.
- Vary the **bread.**
- May use **butter** to fry the sandwich.
- Add canned, chopped, drained green chilies.
- Add **roasted red peppers,** drained and chopped.
- Add **mustard spread** to bread before adding cheese.

ROASTED VEGETABLE SANDWICH

Prep time: 15 minutes
Cook time: 25 minutes

1 serving

Ingredients

1½ ounces broccoli florets
1 carrot, cut into small pieces
½ cup cubed eggplant
2 tablespoons mushrooms
Vegetable oil spray

½ teaspoon thyme
1 teaspoon olive oil
1 tablespoon wine vinegar
Pita bread

Instructions

1. Heat the oven to 350°.
2. Put broccoli, carrots, eggplant, and mushrooms into a baking dish.
3. Spray the vegetables with vegetable oil spray.
4. Sprinkle thyme on the vegetables.
5. Cook about 25 minutes until the vegetables are soft.
6. Mix the oil and vinegar with the vegetables.
7. Put the mixture into the pita pocket.

Nutrient Content

Calories 267
Protein 8 gm
12% calories from Protein
Carbohydrates 46 gm
Fat 6 gm

19% calories from Fat
Cholesterol 0 mg
Sodium 352 mg
Dietary Fiber 6 gm

Adaptations for Physical Limitations

- Adjust the consistency to the swallowing ability of the client by cutting vegetables into small pieces. May not be appropriate for all clients.

Substitutions

- Any combination of **vegetables** may be used.
- Any type of **pita** may be used.
- Sprinkle with 1 teaspoon **grated cheese**.

TURKEY AND CHEESE ROLL-UP

Prep time: 5 minutes
Cook time: None

1 serving

Ingredients

1 tortilla
1 teaspoon mayonnaise
1 teaspoon ketchup
1 leaf lettuce
1 thin slice tomato
1 thin slice onion
2 ounces turkey breast, sliced thin
1 slice Swiss cheese

Instructions

1. Spread the mayonnaise and ketchup over the tortilla.
2. Stack the remainder of the ingredients on the tortilla.
3. Carefully roll it up.
4. Cut into thirds on the diagonal.

Nutrient Content

Calories 373
Protein 24 gm
25% calories from Protein
Carbohydrates 32 gm
Fat 18 gm
41% calories from Fat
Cholesterol 49 mg
Sodium 709 mg
Dietary Fiber .5 gm

Adaptations for Physical Limitations

- Adjust the consistency to the swallowing ability of the client by cutting the tortilla into small pieces.

Substitutions

- Omit the onion or tomato.
- Spread **mustard** on the tortilla in addition to or instead of the **mayonnaise** and **ketchup.**

CHAPTER 22
Recipes for Beverages

Introduction

*Beverages are important. They help with digestion and contribute to the general enjoyment of the meal. Therefore, when served with the meal, they should **compliment** the food. Some people always drink water with their meal. Others drink soda or iced tea. Some drink juice or coffee. Some people drink a cold drink with the meal and a hot beverage such as coffee or tea after the food is finished. Some people like cold drinks; some people like hot ones. Some people like ice in their drinks and some do not. Respect the traditions, cultural preferences, and the practices of the home and the client.*

Beverages are a very good vehicle for increasing the caloric and nutritional intake of a client. They can be served as a snack and as an addition to the meal.

- When offering beverages, take into account any fluid restrictions that may be prescribed.
- Not all beverages are appropriate for all types of diets or restrictions.
- All beverages and fluids must be counted into the daily caloric intake of the client.
- If the client is counting his fluid intake, be sure to count only the fluid actually consumed, not the fluid served.

Recipes included in this chapter:

- Blended Banana
- Café Au Lait

- Creamsicle
- Enriched Iced Coffee
- Fruit Freeze
- Hot Apple Cider
- Vanilla Milkshake
- Strawberry Milk Smoothie
- Yogurt Smoothie

BLENDED BANANA

Prep time: 5 minutes *2 servings*

Ingredients

1 cup skim milk
1 teaspoon vanilla extract

1 small banana, approximately 6–7 inches long, peeled and cut up

Instructions

1. Place all ingredients in a blender and cover.
2. Blend until smooth.
3. Pour into two glasses or dessert dishes.
4. Serve immediately or freeze for dessert.

Nutrient Content

Calories 95
Protein 5 gm
20% calories from Protein
Carbohydrates 18 gm
Fat .5 gm

4% calories from Fat
Cholesterol 2 mg
Sodium 64 mg
Dietary Fiber 1.2 gm

Adaptations for Physical Limitations

- Adjust the consistency to the swallowing ability of the client by blending longer or adding additional liquid.

Substitutions

- Any kind of ***milk*** can be used, including ***chocolate***.
- Cold ***coffee*** may be used instead of milk.
- Imitation vanilla can be used in place of extract.
- $\frac{1}{2}$ cup ***strawberries*** can be added or used in place of banana.

CAFÉ AU LAIT

Prep time: 5 minutes
Cook time: 5 minutes

2 servings

Ingredients

1 cup coffee regular
1 cup milk regular

$\frac{1}{2}$ teaspoon cinnamon (optional)

Instructions

Hot drink
1. Prepare one cup of coffee.
2. Pour coffee into a cup so that the cup is only half full.
3. Warm one cup of milk to the scalding point.
4. Combine the coffee and the milk and serve.
5. Cinnamon can be sprinkled on the top.

Cold drink
1. Prepare one cup of coffee.
2. Pour coffee into a glass so that the glass is only half full. Add ice if preferred.
3. Combine the coffee and cold milk.
4. Cinnamon can be sprinkled on top.

Nutrient Content

Calories 82
Protein 4 gm
20% calories from Protein
Carbohydrates 6 gm
Fat .5 gm

48% calories from Fat
Cholesterol 17 mg
Sodium 62 mg
Dietary Fiber 0 gm

Adaptations for Physical Limitations

- Adjust the consistency to the swallowing ability of the client by adding additional liquid or thickening agent.

Substitutions

- Any coffee can be used, flavored or decaffeinated.
- Any **milk** can be used, including **chocolate** or **skim.**
- Could be served hot or cold over ice.
- **Whipped cream** can be added.

CREAMSICLE

Prep time: 5 minutes *1 serving*

Ingredients

1 cup low fat 1% milk   1 cup orange sherbet

Instructions

1. Mix or blend milk and orange sherbet until smooth
2. Serve immediately

Nutrient Content

Calories 323
Protein 11 gm
14% calories from Protein
Carbohydrates 58.5 gm
Fat 6 gm

16% calories from Fat
Cholesterol 19 mg
Sodium 211.5 mg
Dietary Fiber 0 gm

Adaptations for Physical Limitations

- Adjust the consistency to the swallowing ability of the client by blending longer or adding additional liquid or thickening agent.

Substitutions

- Any *milk* may be used.
- Any flavor *sherbet* may be used.
- Serve over crushed ice.

ENRICHED ICED COFFEE

Prep time: 5 minutes *1 serving*

Ingredients

1 cup coffee, cooled
3 tablespoon nonfat dry milk
½ cup vanilla ice cream

2 tablespoon whipped topping (optional)
6 ice cubes

Instructions

1. Place coffee, nonfat dry milk, and ice cubes in a blender and cover.
2. Blend until semismooth.
3. Add ice cream.
4. Blend another 10–15 seconds.
5. Pour into glass.
6. Top with whipped topping.
7. Serve immediately.

Nutrient Content

Calories 234
Protein 11 gm
18% calories from Protein
Carbohydrates 29 gm
Fat 9 gm

33% calories from Fat
Cholesterol 38 mg
Sodium 190 mg
Dietary Fiber 0 gm

Adaptations for Physical Limitations

- Adjust the consistency to the swallowing ability of the client by blending longer or adding additional liquid or thickening agent.

Substitutions

- Any coffee may be used, flavored or decaffeinated.
- *Frozen yogurt* or *ice milk* may be used.
- Any *milk* can be used, including chocolate.
- *Whipped cream* may be used in place of whipped topping.

FRUIT FREEZE

Prep time: 5 minutes *3 servings*

Ingredients

1½ cups orange juice
1 cup frozen, unsweetened strawberries

½ cup low-fat lemon yogurt
2 teaspoons honey (optional)

Instructions

1. Place all ingredients in a blender and cover.
2. Blend until mixture is smooth and creamy.
3. Pour into glass.
4. Serve immediately.

Nutrient Content

Calories 130
Protein 3 gm
9% calories from Protein
Carbohydrates 29 gm
Fat 1 gm

7% calories from Fat
Cholesterol 2 mg
Sodium 30 mg
Dietary Fiber 2 gm

Adaptations for Physical Limitations

- Adjust the consistency to the swallowing ability of the client by blending longer or adding additional liquid or thickening agent.

Substitutions

- Any berries can used in place of strawberries.
- **Vanilla or fruited yogurt** can be used in place of lemon.

HOT APPLE CIDER

Prep time: 5 minutes
Cook time: 5 minutes

1 serving

Ingredients

1 cup apple cider
1 whole clove or ½ teaspoon ground
1 cinnamon stick or ½ teaspoon cinnamon powder

2 orange slices

Instructions

1. Warm the apple cider.
2. Add the clove, cinnamon, and orange.
3. Simmer 3 minutes.
4. Pour into a cup and drink.

Nutrient Content

Calories 155
Protein .68 gm
2% calories from Protein
Carbohydrates 36 gm
Fat .3 gm

2% calories from Fat
Cholesterol 0 mg
Sodium 2 mg
Dietary Fiber 2 gm

Adaptations for Physical Limitations

- Adjust the consistency to the swallowing ability of the client by adding additional liquid or a thickening agent.

Substitutions

- *Apple juice* can be used in place of apple cider.

STRAWBERRY MILK SMOOTHIE

Prep time: 5 minutes   *2 servings*

Ingredients

1 cup skim milk
¾ cup sliced strawberries
1 teaspoon vanilla extract
1 teaspoon lemon juice

Instructions

1. Place all ingredients into a blender and cover.
2. Blend at high speed until smooth.
3. Pour into two glasses and serve.

Nutrient Content

Calories 68
Protein 4.5 gm
28% calories from Protein
Carbohydrates 11 gm
Fat .5 gm
6% calories from Fat
Cholesterol 2 mg
Sodium 64 mg
Dietary Fiber 1.4 gm

Adaptations for Physical Limitations

- Adjust the consistency to the swallowing ability of the client by blending longer or adding additional liquid or thickening agent.

Substitutions

- Any *milk* can be used instead of chocolate.
- Imitation vanilla can be used in place of vanilla extract.
- Almond extract can be used in place of vanilla extract.
- Ice may be placed in the glass before pouring in the liquid.

VANILLA MILKSHAKE

Prep time: 5 minutes   *1 serving*

Ingredients

1 cup milk
½ cup vanilla ice cream

Whipped cream or whipped topping (optional)

Instructions

1. Mix ingredients in a blender until smooth.
2. Serve immediately.
3. Discard any unused portion.

Nutrient Content

Calories 283
Protein 10 gm
14% calories from Protein
Carbohydrates 27 gm
Fat 15 gm

48% calories from Fat
Cholesterol 62 mg
Sodium 172 mg
Dietary Fiber 0 gm

Adaptations for Physical Limitations

- Adjust the consistency to the swallowing ability of the client by blending longer or adding additional liquid or thickening agent.

Substitutions

- Any flavored *ice cream, ice milk,* or *frozen yogurt* can be used.
- Any *milk* can be used, including *skim* or *chocolate.*
- *Liquid ice cream sauces* (toppings) can be used to change the flavor.

YOGURT SMOOTHIE

Prep time: 5 minutes *3 servings*

Ingredients

1½ cups low fat vanilla yogurt
1 small banana
1 tablespoon orange juice concentrate

¾ cup frozen peaches.
1 cup frozen whole strawberries
3 ice cubes

Instructions

1. Place all ingredients in a blender and cover.
2. Blend at high speed for 30 seconds or until smooth.
3. Pour into glass.
4. Serve immediately.

Nutrient Content

Calories 202
Protein 8 gm
14% calories from Protein
Carbohydrates 40 gm
Fat 2 gm

9% calories from Fat
Cholesterol 7.5 mg
Sodium 92 mg
Dietary Fiber 3.5 gm

Adaptations for Physical Limitations

- Adjust the consistency to the swallowing ability of the client by blending longer or adding additional liquid or thickening agent.

Substitutions

- Any kind of **vanilla yogurt** can be used.
- Serve with **whipped topping** if desired.

CHAPTER 23

Recipes for Snacks

Introduction

Snacks are an important part of the daily diet. They offer variety and provide a way to eat small amounts of foods and to enjoy one single food. They often provide additional calories and nutrients that are not consumed at mealtimes. Snacks are often part of another activity such as watching television, visiting with friends, or preparing for bed.

When reviewing the daily nutritional intake of your client, be sure to allow for snacks. Discuss these snacks with your client. Snacks should be things your client looks forward to. Snacks and the enjoyment they give are individual. Respect your client's preferences.

Recipes included in this chapter:

- Apple Crisp
- Blueberry Muffins
- Bran Muffins
- Corn Bread
- Fritters
- Fruity Spread for Graham Crackers
- Raisin Oatmeal Bars
- Rice Pudding

APPLE CRISP

Prep time: 20 minutes
Cook time: 30 minutes

8 servings

Ingredients

4 cups sliced tart apples (about 4 medium apples)
$2/3$ cup light brown sugar packed
$1/2$ cup all-purpose flour
$1/2$ cup quick-cooking oats (uncooked)

$3/4$ teaspoon cinnamon
$3/4$ teaspoon nutmeg
$1/3$ cup butter or margarine, softened
Vegetable oil spray

Instructions

1. Preheat oven to 375°.
2. Spray 8- or 9-inch square pan with vegetable oil spray.
3. Place apples in pan.
4. Mix remaining ingredients thoroughly.
5. Sprinkle over apples.
6. Bake 30 minutes or until apples are tender and top is golden brown.
7. Serve warm if desired.

Nutrient Content

Calories 221
Protein 2 gm
3% calories from Protein
Carbohydrates 37 gm
Fat 8 gm

33% calories from Fat
Cholesterol 21 mg
Sodium 86 mg
Dietary Fiber 3 gm

Adaptations for Physical Limitations

- Adjust the consistency to the swallowing ability of the client by cutting the servings into small pieces.

Substitutions

- Top with $1/3$ cup ground **nuts** of choice.
- Serve with *ice cream, yogurt,* or *frozen dessert topping.*

BLUEBERRY MUFFINS

Prep time: 5 minutes
Cook time: 25 minutes

12 muffins

Ingredients

1 large egg
1 cup milk
¼ cup vegetable oil
2 cups all-purpose flour
¼ cup sugar

3 teaspoons baking powder
1 teaspoon salt
¾ cup well-drained frozen unsweetened blueberries, thawed
Vegetable oil spray

Instructions

1. Heat oven to 400°.
2. Spray bottoms of 12 medium muffin cups with vegetable oil spray.
3. Beat egg; stir in milk and oil.
4. Mix in flour, sugar, baking powder, and salt until flour is just moistened.
5. Batter will be lumpy.
6. Fold in blueberries.
7. Fill muffin cups ⅔ full.
8. Bake 20–25 minutes or until golden brown.
9. Test by inserting a toothpick into the center of a muffin. It is done if the toothpick comes out clean.
10. Remove from pan immediately.
11. Serve.

Nutrient Content

Calories 151
Protein 3 gm
8% calories from Protein
Carbohydrates 23 gm
Fat 5 gm

32% calories from Fat
Cholesterol 3 mg
Sodium 331 mg
Dietary Fiber 1 gm

Adaptations for Physical Limitations

- Adjust the consistency to the swallowing ability of the client by cutting the blueberries before using them. Cut the muffins into small pieces.

Substitutions

- 1 cup fresh **blueberries** may be used in place of frozen.
- Any **berries** may be used.
- Use **skim milk**.

BRAN MUFFINS

Prep time: 10 minutes
Cook time: 25 minutes

12 muffins

Ingredients

1 cup all-purpose flour
1 cup bran cereal
¼ cup wheat germ
2½ teaspoons baking powder
½ teaspoon salt

1 medium egg
2 tablespoons margarine or butter
¼ cup molasses
¾ cup skim milk
Vegetable oil spray

Instructions

1. Preheat oven to 400°.
2. Grease 12 medium muffin cups.
3. Stir together flour, bran cereal, wheat germ, baking powder, and salt into a medium bowl. Set aside.
4. Mix egg, margarine, molasses, and milk in blender or food processor. Blend until smooth.
5. Pour milk mixture onto the flour mixture and mix just until flour is moistened. Batter will be lumpy.
6. Pour batter into each muffin tin.
7. Bake for 20–25 minutes
8. Test by inserting a toothpick into the center of a muffin. It is done if the toothpick it comes out clean
9. Remove muffins immediately from cups.

Nutrient Content

Calories 122
Protein 4 gm
13% calories from Protein
Carbohydrates 22 gm
Fat 3 gm

21% calories from Fat
Cholesterol 16 mg
Sodium 267 mg
Dietary Fiber 3 gm

Adaptations for Physical Limitations

- Adjust the consistency to the swallowing ability of the client by cutting the muffins into small pieces.

Substitutions

- Use **_whole milk_** instead of skim milk.
- Add ½ cup **_raisins._**

CORN BREAD

Prep time: 10 minutes
Cook time: 25 minutes

9 servings

Ingredients

1 cup yellow cornmeal
1 cup all-purpose flour
2 tablespoons sugar
4 teaspoons baking powder
$\frac{1}{2}$ teaspoon salt

1 cup whole milk
$\frac{1}{4}$ cup margarine, softened, or shortening
1 large egg
Vegetable oil spray

Instructions

1. Preheat oven to 425°.
2. Spray 8- or 9-inch square pan with vegetable oil spray.
3. Blend all ingredients about 30 seconds.
4. Beat well for 1 minute.
5. Pour into pan.
6. Bake 20–25 minutes or until golden brown.
7. Test by inserting a toothpick into the center of bread. It is done if the toothpick comes out clean.
8. Cut into 2-inch pieces.

Nutrient Content

Calories 178
Protein 4 gm
9% calories from Protein
Carbohydrates 25 gm
Fat 7 gm

36% calories from Fat
Cholesterol 27 mg
Sodium 475 mg
Dietary Fiber 1 gm

Adaptations for Physical Limitations

- Adjust the consistency to the swallowing ability of the client by cutting the corn bread into small pieces.

Substitutions

- Use *skim milk* instead of whole milk.
- Serve with *butter* or *margarine* or *jelly.*

FRITTERS

Prep time: 10 minutes
Cook time: 5 minutes

4 servings

Ingredients

1 cup all-purpose flour
1 teaspoon baking powder
1 teaspoon salt
Fat of frying

2 large eggs
$\frac{1}{2}$ cup milk
1 teaspoon vegetable oil

Instructions

1. Heat oil (3 to 4 inches) to 375° in deep fat fryer or pot.
2. Mix all ingredients well in a bowl.
3. Drop level tablespoonfuls into hot fat and fry about 5 minutes or until thoroughly cooked.
4. Drain and serve.

Nutrient Content

Calories 180
Protein 7 gm
17% calories from Protein
Carbohydrates 26 gm
Fat 5 gm

25% calories from Fat
Cholesterol 110 mg
Sodium 719 mg
Dietary Fiber 0 gm

Adaptations for Physical Limitations

- Adjust the consistency to the swallowing ability of the client by mashing fritter with fork or cutting into small pieces. Puree in blender with additional liquid if needed.

Substitutions

- If desired, stir about 1 cup of cooked *corn,* chopped *apple, banana,* cooked cubed *meats,* or cooked *shrimp* into fritter batter.

FRUITY SPREAD FOR GRAHAM CRACKERS

Prep time: 10 minutes
Cook time: None

5 servings

Ingredients

1 finely chopped medium apple, peeled
1 tablespoon lemon juice
8 ounces nonfat cream cheese
2 tablespoons sugar
1 teaspoon cinnamon

½ cup raisins
1 carrot, peeled and shredded (about ¼ cup)
16 graham cracker squares

Instructions

1. Mix apples with lemon juice to prevent browning. Set aside.
2. Mix cream cheese, sugar, and cinnamon well with a mixer if possible.
3. Add raisins, carrots, and apple. Mix well.
4. Spread on graham crackers or bread of choice.
5. Store spread tightly covered in refrigerator for up to 4 days.

Nutrient Content

Calories 183
Protein 8 gm
17% calories from Protein
Carbohydrates 34 gm
Fat 2 gm

11% calories from Fat
Cholesterol 4 mg
Sodium 320 mg
Dietary Fiber 2 gm

Adaptations for Physical Limitations

- Adjust the consistency to the swallowing ability of the client by mashing the crackers with a fork.

Substitutions

- Any *jelly* or *jam* or all *fruit spread* can be used.
- Any variety of *cracker* can be used.
- Use 2 tablespoons creamy *peanut butter* in place of fruity spread.
- Use *toast, bagels,* or *bread* for the spread.
- Use regular *cream cheese.*

RAISIN OATMEAL BARS

Prep time: 20 minutes
Cook time: 30 minutes

16 servings

Ingredients

¾ cup packed brown sugar
½ cup sugar
4 tablespoons margarine, softened
¾ cup unsweetened applesauce
2 egg whites
2 tablespoons skim milk

2 teaspoons vanilla
1½ cups all-purpose flour
1 teaspoon baking soda
1 teaspoon cinnamon
3 cups quick oats, uncooked
1 cup raisins

Instructions

1. Preheat oven to 350°.
2. Mix or beat sugars and margarine well.
3. Add applesauce, egg whites, milk, and vanilla. Beat well.
4. Slowly add flour, baking soda, and cinnamon. Mix well.
5. Stir in oats and raisins. Mix well.
6. Spread dough in ungreased 13 × 9 baking pan.
7. Bake 25–30 minutes or until light brown.
8. Cool before cutting into bars.
9. Cut into 16 bars.
10. Serve.

Nutrient Content

Calories 189
Protein 4 gm
8% calories from Protein
Carbohydrates 35 gm
Fat 4 gm

18% calories from Fat
Cholesterol 0 mg
Sodium 126 mg
Dietary Fiber 2 gm

Adaptations for Physical Limitations

- Adjust the consistency to the swallowing ability of the client by moistened with liquid. May not be appropriate for all clients.

Substitutions

- Use **butter** in place of margarine.
- Use **whole milk** in place of skim.
- Use uncooked old-fashioned **oats** in place of quick oats.
- Add ½ cup chopped **nuts**.

RICE PUDDING

Prep time: 5 minutes
Cook time: 20 minutes

3 servings

Ingredients

1 tablespoon cornstarch
1½ tablespoon sugar
1 medium egg, slightly beaten
1 cup milk

½ cup cooked rice
½ teaspoon vanilla
Sprinkle cinnamon

Instructions

1. In saucepan, blend cornstarch, sugar, and egg until smooth.
2. Add milk slowly, stirring to mix well.
3. Add rice.
4. Cook over medium heat until mixture is thick and comes to a boil.
5. Remove from heat, add vanilla, and cool.
6. Sprinkle with cinnamon.
7. May serve warm or chill for 1 hour.

Nutrient Content

Calories 149
Protein 5 gm
14% calories from Protein
Carbohydrates 22 gm
Fat 4 gm

26% calories from Fat
Cholesterol 73 mg
Sodium 59 mg
Dietary Fiber 0 gm

Adaptations for Physical Limitations

- Adjust the consistency to the swallowing ability of the client by pureeing after cooking.

Substitutions

- Sprinkle with nutmeg in place of or in addition to cinnamon.
- May use *skim milk* in place of milk.

Appendix

Table A Common Substitutions

- Vegetable oil spray can always be substituted for oil or butter when browning, sautéing or pan-frying food.
- $1/2$ cup pasta can be added to any soup.
- Egg substitute can be used instead of an egg when breading meat, poultry, or chicken.
- Seasoned or plain breadcrumbs can usually be used interchangeably. Seasoned breadcrumbs have spices and may contain sodium, so take this into consideration when spicing the dish or following a dietary restriction.
- Olive oil, vegetable oil, canola oil, and safflower oil are interchangeable. Peanut oil adds a distinct flavor and should be used only if that flavor is wanted.
- 1 tablespoon of fresh herbs = 1 teaspoon of dried herbs
- 1 medium onion = $1/2$ cup chopped onion
- 1 medium lemon = 3 tablespoons lemon juice
- 1 medium carrot = $1/2$ cup chopped carrot
- 1 small clove garlic = $1/8$ teaspoon garlic powder
- 1 cup brown sugar = $3/4$ cup white granulated sugar + $1/4$ cup molasses
- 1 cup white granulated sugar = 1 cup firmly packed brown sugar
- To make buttermilk, add 1 tablespoon of lemon juice or white vinegar to 1 cup of milk or yogurt. Let stand 5 minutes. Use immediately.
- Use yogurt instead of sour cream in soups and all cooking.
- Fat-free milk can be substituted for regular milk in most recipes.

Table B Terms Used in Recipes for Preparing, Cooking, or Combining Ingredients

Word	Definition
Baste	To put a liquid onto foods as they are cooking
Beat	To make mixture smooth by mixing with spoon, whip, or beater
Blend	To thoroughly combine all ingredients until very smooth and uniform
Boil	To heat until bubbles rise continuously and break on the surface of the liquid
Brown	To cook until food changes color to brown
Chill	To refrigerate, to make cold
Chop	To cut into small pieces
Cool	To allow food to get to a lower temperature
Crush	To press to extract juice with garlic press, mallet, or side of knife
Cube	To cut into squares $1/2$ inch or larger
Dice	To cut into small cubes usually less than $1/2$ inch
Drain	To separate the liquid and the solid part of a food substance
Fry	To cook food in fat
Grate	To cut into tiny particles by rubbing the food over the holes of a grater
Grill	To cook food directly over a heat source
Julienne	To cut into long thin stips
Legumes	Vegetables that bear their fruit or seeds in pods (peas, beans, lentils)
Marinate	To let food stand in liquid that will add flavor or tenderize
Mince	To cut into very small pieces
Mix	To combine in any way that distributes all ingredients evenly
Peel	To strip off outer covering
Picked over	To go through food so as to remove debris, shells, or inedible particles
Refrigerate	Place in refrigerator to store
Roasted	To cook with hot air, usually in an oven
Sauté	To cook in a shallow pan with a small amount of fat
Scoop	To remove something with a spoon or ladle
Shred	To cut into thin pieces using large holes on grater or shredder
Simmer	To cook in liquid just below the boiling point
Sliver	To cut into long thin pieces
Snip	To cut into very small pieces with scissors
Sprinkle	To spread a liquid or any fine substance on the surface of another
Steam	To cook over a liquid without submerging the food
Stir	To combine ingredients with circular or figure 8 motion until uniform consistency
Toast	To brown in oven or toaster
Whip	To beat rapidly in order to incorporate air into the food

Table C Nutrient Content of Food Items

Item	Serving Size	Calories (kcals)	PRO gm	% from PRO	CHO gm	Fat	% from Fat	Chol mg	Sodium mg	Dietary Fiber gm
Almonds, toasted	1 teaspoon	14	0.5	13	0.5	1.25	74	0	0	0.25
Bacon bits	1 teaspoon	10	1	40	0	0.67	60	0	104	0
Bacon, strip, crisp	1 strip	36	2	8	—	3	77	5.3	101	0
Beef, ground, extra lean, raw	1 ounce	66	5	34	0	5	66	19	19	0
Blueberries, frozen	½ cup	40	—	3	9	—	11	0	1	2
Blueberries, fresh	½ cup	56	0.67	4	14	0.3	6	0	6	2.7
Butter	1 tablespoon	101	—	—	—	11.5	99	31	117	0
Carrots, raw	½ cup	27.5	0.6	9	6	—	4	0	22	2
Celery, raw	½ cup	10	0.4	11	2	—	8	0	52	1
Cheese, American	1 ounce	106	6	25	0.5	9	73	27	184	0
Cheese, cheddar	1 ounce	114	7	26	—	9	72	30	176	0
Cheese, grated Parmesan	1 tablespoon	23	2	39	—	1.5	58	4	93	0

continues

Table C *(continued)*

Item	Serving Size	Calories (kcals)	PRO gm	% from PRO	CHO gm	Fat	% from Fat	Chol mg	Sodium mg	Dietary Fiber gm
Cheese, mozzarella, part skim	1 ounce	72	7	41	1	5	55	16	132	0
Cheese, Swiss	1 ounce	107	8	32	1	8	64	26	74	0
Chicken breast, grilled, no skin	3 ounces	140	26	80	0	3	19.5	72	63	0
Cinnamon	½ teaspoon	3	—	—	1	—	—	0	—	—
Cottage cheese, creamed	¼ cup	54	6.5	52	1	2	38	8	213	0
Cottage cheese, nonfat	¼ cup	31	6	87	1	—	4	2	5	0
Egg, large, hard boiled	1 egg	78	6	35	0.5	5	48	212	62	0
Eggs, liquid	¼ cup	53	7.5	62	—	2	35	1	111	0
Fruit, dried mixed	1 ounce	69	.7	3	18	—	1.7	0	5	2
Half and half	¼ cup	79	2	10	3	7	78	22	25	0
Honey	1 tablespoon	64	—	—	17	0	0	0	0.8	—
Ice Cream, vanilla	½ cup	133	2	7	15.5	7	48	29	53	0
Jelly, grape	1 tablespoon	54	—	—	13	—	—	0	5	—
Jelly, mint	1 tablespoon	54	0	0	12	0	0	0	0	0

Juice, apple	½ cup	54	0	0	13	0	0	0	7	0
Juice, orange	½ cup	55	1	6	13	—	5	0	1	—
Ketchup	1 tablespoon	16	—	3	4	—	3	0	178	—
Margarine	1 tablespoon	101	—	—	—	11	99	0	133	0
Marmalade, orange	1 tablespoon	49	—	—	13	0	0	0	11	—
Mayonnaise	1 tablespoon	100	0	0	0	11	100	5	80	0
Mayonnaise, low fat	1 tablespoon	25	0	0	4	1	36	0	140	0
Milk, 1%	½ cup	51	4	34	6	1	22	5	62	0
Milk, 2%	½ cup	98	5	30	7	2	31	9	72	0
Milk, skim	½ cup	43	4	42	6	—	5	2	64	0
Milk, whole	½ cup	75	4	23	6	4	48	17	60	0
Mushrooms	½ cup	9	1	30	1	—	11	0	1	—
Mustard, yellow	1 teaspoon	3							56	
Noodles, cooked	½ cup	106	4	14	20	1	9	26	6	—
Nuts, peanuts	1 tablespoon	36	2	15	2	2	58	0	84	1
Nuts, walnuts, chopped	1 tablespoon									
Oil, vegetable	1 tablespoon	120	0	0	0	14	100	0	0	0
Olives	½ cup	77	0.5	2	4	7	78	0	586	2

continues

Table C *(continued)*

Item	Serving Size	Calories (kcals)	PRO gm	% from PRO	CHO gm	Fat	% from Fat	Chol mg	Sodium mg	Dietary Fiber gm
Onions, raw, chopped	¼ cup	15	0.5	8	3	—	4	0	1	1
Peanut butter, creamy	1 tablespoon	95	4	15	3	8	72	0	75	1
Pepper, black, ground	1 teaspoon	5	—							
Peppers, green	½ cup	20	1	8	5	—	6	0	1	1
Preserves, apricot	1 tablespoon	48	—	1	13	—	—	0	8	—
Raisins	1 tablespoon	27	—	4	7	—	1	0	1	—
Rice, brown, cooked	½ cup	109	2	8	23	1	7	0	1	2
Rice, white, cooked	½ cup	121	2	7	27	0	1	—	0	0
Salt, table	1 teaspoon	0	0	0	0	0	0	0	2325	0
Sausage	1 ounce	98	4	18	—	9	82	22	207	0
Sour cream	1 tablespoon	31	0.5	6	1	3	86	6	8	0
Soy sauce	1 teaspoon	2							341	
Sugar, brown	1 tablespoon	36	0	0	9	0	0	0	4	0
Sugar, white	1 tablespoon	49	0	0	13	0	0	0	—	0

Tomatoes, stewed, no salt, canned	15 ounces	118	—	10	30	0	0	0	169	7
Turkey, ground	1/2 cup	170	20	50	0	9	50	90	107	0
Unsweetened, frozen blueberry	1/2 cup	39.5	0.3	2.7	9	0.5	10.5	0	0.77	2
Vinegar, wine	1/2 cup	0	0	0	0	0	0	0	0	0
Whipped cream topping	1/2 cup	77	1	5	4	7	76	23	39	0
Yogurt, plain, skim milk	1/2 cup	63	6	44	9	—	3	2	86	0
Yogurt, plain, whole milk	1/2 cup	69	4	24	5	4	47	14	54	0
Yogurt, vanilla, low fat	1/2 cup	97	5.5	26	15.5	1	13	5.5	74	0
Zucchini, raw, uncooked	1/2 cup	8	1	27	2	—	7	0	2	1

Table D Seasonings Common to Cultural Groups

Group	Seasonings
Cajun	Chilies, hot sauce
Caribbean	Allspice, ginger, jerk, lime, chilies, cilantro, cinnamon, cloves, curry, garlic, mace, nutmeg, pepper, sugar, vanilla
Chinese	Cilantro, crushed red pepper, basil, cardamom, garlic, ginger, five spice powder (anise, Szechwan pepper, fennel, cloves, cinnamon) hoisin, sesame, sesame seeds, star anise, Szechwan pepper, whole red chilies
Greek	Cinnamon, dill, garlic, licorice, mint, oregano, paprika
Indian	Anise, cardamom, cassia, chili, cinnamon, cloves, coriander, curry, cumin, dill, fennel, garlic, ginger, lemon, nutmeg, mace, mint, pepper, poppy seeds, saffron, sesame, tamarind, turmeric
Italian	Anise, basil, crushed red pepper, fennel, garlic, oregano, parsley, rosemary, sage
Latin American	Black pepper, curry, saffron
Mexican	Cayenne, chili powder, cilantro, cinnamon, cumin, garlic, jalapeno peppers, lime, pepper, vanilla
Middle East	Allspice, anise, candied peel, chilies, cilantro, cinnamon, cloves, coriander, fennel, garlic, honey, parsley, poppy seeds, saffron, sesame
Portuguese	Chilies, cilantro, garlic
Russian	Caraway seeds, cinnamon, dill, clove, coriander, parsley, nutmeg
Scandinavian	Cardamom, dill, mustard
Spanish	Capers, chilies, cinnamon, coriander, cumin, garlic, paprika, parsley, pepper, saffron, turmeric, vanilla
Thai	Basil, cardamom, chilies, cilantro, cinnamon, coriander, cumin, curry, garlic, ginger, lemongrass, lime, mint, red chilies, red pepper, tamarind, turmeric
Vietnamese	Basil, chilies, cilantro, garlic, ginger, lemon, lemongrass, lime, mint, star anise

Table E Equivalent Measures

Common Measure Equivalents

1 teaspoon = $\frac{1}{2}$ tablespoon
3 teaspoons = 1 tablespoon
2 tablespoons = 1 ounce
16 tablespoons = 1 cup
1 cup = $\frac{1}{2}$ pint
2 cups = 1 pint
4 cups = 1 quart
2 pints = 1 quart
4 quarts (liquid) = 1 gallon
4 tablespoons = $\frac{1}{4}$ cup
$5\frac{1}{3}$ tablespoon = $\frac{1}{3}$ cup

Metric Equivalents

Volume
$\frac{1}{4}$ teaspoon = 1.5 ml
$\frac{1}{2}$ teaspoon = 3 ml
1 teaspoon = 5 ml
1 tablespoon = 15 ml
$\frac{1}{4}$ cup = 60 ml
$\frac{1}{2}$ cup = 125 ml
$\frac{3}{4}$ cup = 180 ml
1 cup = 250 ml
2 cups = 500 ml
3 cups = 750 ml

Weight
1 ounce = 28 grams
$\frac{1}{2}$ pound = 225 grams
1 pound = 450 grams
16 ounces = 450 grams

Oven Temperatures

300° F = 149° C
350° F = 175° C
375° F = 190° C
450° F = 230° C

Glossary

Chapter	Word	Definition
1	nutritious	Substances that promote nutrition
1	nutrient	Food substances that are required by the body to repair, maintain, and grow new cells
1	lifecycle	The complete series of events during a person's existence
1	supplements	Substances taken in addition to food
1	health care professional	A person credentialed by a recognized body to give health-related information and activities
1	carbohydrates	One of the basic food elements necessary for the body to function properly; includes all sugars and starches
1	complex	Referring to many sugars linked together to form a long chain
1	simple	Referring to single and double sugar molecules
1	proteins	One of the nutrients necessary to all animal life
1	enzymes	Protein catalysts supplied by the body and necessary to utilize nutrients
1	hormones	Protein substances secreted by an endocrine gland directly into the bloodstream
1	essential amino acids	Proteins that the body must have to function properly
1	antibodies	Substances in the body that fight disease
1	synthesized	To combine and make a more complex new product
1	fat	Soft, solid, semisolid, or liquid compound; one of the three main nutrients
1	essential fatty acids	Polyunsaturated fatty acids that are necessary and must be provided through the diet
1	saturated fats	Fats derived from animal and dairy sources
1	cholesterol	A fat both ingested and produced by the body
1	unsaturated fat	A fat that is liquid at room temperature
1	hydrogenation	A process by which fat is hardened
1	calories	Unit for measuring the energy produced when food is oxidized in the body
1	vitamins	Organic substances derived from plants and animals necessary in small amounts for the body to function
1	minerals	Inorganic substances necessary in small amounts for the body to function
1	micronutrients	Nutrients necessary in small amounts
1	basic food groups	Food that gives similar nutrients

Chapter	Word	Definition
1	pyramid	A display that presents the ideal number of servings of each food group
1	moderation	In small amounts
1	prescribed diet	An individualized plan of eating created by a health care professional to meet an identified need
1	physical activity	Involving bodily movements or activity exerting muscles in various ways
1	sodium	One of the elements of salt
1	sodium chloride	Salt
1	alcohol	The intoxicating part of liquid formed from fermented sugars
1	vegetarians	Those who eat vegetables and vegetable products
1	vegan	Those who eat vegetables and vegetable products
1	Lacto-vegetarian	Those who eat dairy and plants
1	Ovo-vegetarian	Those who eat eggs and plants
1	Lacto-ovo-vegetarian	Those who eat dairy, eggs, and plants
1	semi-vegetarian	Those who exclude red meat from their diet
1	therapeutic diet	Medically needed diet used in the science of healing
2	dietary supplements	Substances that increase the nutritional value of a diet
2	chronic	State of disease that lasts a long time
2	acute	State of disease that comes on suddenly and may be of short duration
2	herbs	A plant whose stems are soft and perishable and that has some usefulnes to man either in cooking or as a medicinal supplement
2	phytochemicals	Substances that are derived from plants
2	antioxidants	Substances that prevent or retard the combining of substances with oxygen
2	oxidation	Combining of a substance with oxygen
3	age appropriate	An action or item that is related positively to age and status of the client
3	assistive devices	Mechanical items used to help a person complete a task
3	unaffected side	The side or limb of the body that is not impaired by disease or injury
3	numb	Having no feeling due to lack of circulation
4	culture	The rules and mores a group of people adopt and by which they interact with each other
4	kosher	The rules by which many of those of the Jewish faith slaughter, prepare, and eat food
5	staples	Items usually found in a pantry; a common item used in food preparation
5	brand name	The registered commercial name of a substance or item
6	pasteurized	Heating a food to high temperatures to kill microorganisms

Chapter	Word	Definition
6	unit pricing	A system showing the cost of food in terms of a common measurement such as ounces or pounds
6	convenience food	Edible items partially or wholly commercially prepared and ready to be eaten when purchased
6	reference diet	Diet on which food label analysis is based, usually 2,000 calories
7	microorganisms	Small living things visible only through a microscope
7	permeable	Allowing a substance or organism to pass through
7	freezer burn	The grayish color formed on the edges of frozen food as a result of coming into contact with cold air in the freezer
7	thaw	To convert from a frozen state to a liquid or soft state
7	marinate	To soak a food in a liquid so as to impart flavor and/or tenderize it
7	cross-contamination	Becoming infected from a new or different organism from a new source within the house
8	glucose	Simple form of sugar carried by the blood and used by all tissues
8	milligrams	A unit of measure
8	brine	Salted water used for pickling or preserving food
9	lipid	One of a group of substances including fats and esters
9	body fat	Adipose tissue that is maintained on the body frame
9	dietary lipids	Fat that is found in food
9	cholesterol levels	The amount of cholesterol found in the bloodstream
10	diabetes	Condition that develops when the body cannot change sugar into energy
10	endocrine	A gland secreting a hormone into the bloodstream
10	insulin	Hormone produced by the pancreas and needed for the metabolism of sugars and starches
11	modifications	Changes
11	fiber	An elongated threadlike structure found in food
11	dietary fiber	Fiber that is eaten
11	soluble fiber	Fiber that is eaten and dissolved and absorbed by the body
11	insoluble fiber	Fiber that is eaten and not dissolved and excreted by the body in fecal matter
11	restrict	To limit
11	low-residue, low-fiber diet	Diet that includes eating foods that are low in all kinds of fiber and leave few by-products in the bowel
11	clear liquid diet	Fluids that are clear liquid or liquefy at body temperature, are easily absorbed with little stimulation to the gastrointestinal tract, and leave little or no residue
11	peristalsis	Movement of the intestines that pushes food along to the next part of the intestines
11	full liquid diet	A diet containing those foods that are liquid or liquefy at body temperature
11	lactose	Sugar found in milk products

Chapter	Word	Definition
11	soft diet	Any diet that does not contain items difficult to chew and swallow
11	bland	Low in or devoid of added spice
11	mechanical soft diet	Any diet that does not contain items difficult to chew and swallow
11	pureed diet	Food that is mashed to a smooth consistency
11	blenderized	Food that has been put into a blender and pureed or liquified
11	dysphagia diet	An individualized diet that is safe for a person who has difficultly swallowing
11	commercial thickeners	Substances prepared commercially and added to liquid to provide a more solid consistency
12	absorption	Taking up of fluids, gases, nutrients, or other substances
12	miso	Fermented soybeans
13	edema	Abnormal swelling of a part of the body caused by fluid collecting in that area
13	gas	One of the normal by-products of digestion
13	nausea	The feeling preceeding or leading to vomiting
13	vomiting	Expelling food or partially digested food through the mouth
13	dehydration	Condition in which the body has less than the normal amount of fluid
13	constipation	Having hard, difficult-to-expel bowel movements
13	diarrhea	Abnormally frequent discharge of liquid fecal matter
13	enteral	Nutrition support given by any route that connects to the gastrointestinal tract; can be administered orally or through a tube
13	nasogastric	A tube placed through the nose and the esophagus into the stomach
13	gastrostomy	A tube placed through the skin directly into the stomach
13	jejunostomy	A tube placed through the skin directly into the jejunum of the intestines
13	total parenteral nutrition (TPN)	Nutrition that is given directly into a vein
Intro	analysis	The separation of each recipe into specific nutrient components
Intro	yield	The amount produced

Index

ABCs, 9–11
Acorn squash, baked, 149
Age-appropriate communication, 23, 30
Alcoholic beverages, 10–11, 92
Amino acids, 2
Antacids, 89
Antibiotics, 89
Antibodies, 2
Anticonvulsants, 89
Antidepressants, 90
Antihistamines, 90
Antihypertensives, 90
Antioxidants, 15
Appetite loss, 95–96
Apple cider, hot, 236
Apple crisp, 242
Apples, baked, 185
Aspirin, 90
Assistive devices, 23–24
Asthma medication, 90

Baked acorn squash, 149
Baked apples, 185
Baked fish, 138
Baked potatoes, 166
Balsamic vinaigrette dressing, 216
Banana, blended, 231
Bananas, 78
Barley with mushrooms, 178
Basic food groups, 6–8
Basic lemon dressing, 217
Beans, dry, 8
Bean soup, 105
Beef recipes
　beef stew, 115
　chili, 116
　meatloaf, 117
　pepper steak, 118
　pot roast, 119
　sloppy joes, 120
　tips for, 113–14
Beef stew, 115

Beta-carotene, 15
Beverage recipes
　blended banana, 231
　café au lait, 232
　creamsicle, 233
　enriched iced coffee, 234
　fruit freeze, 235
　hot apple cider, 236
　strawberry milk smoothie, 237
　vanilla milkshake, 238
　yogurt smoothie, 239
Beverages
　alcoholic, 10–11, 92
　types of, 229
Birth control pills, 90
Blended banana, 231
Blenderized foods, 82
Blintzes, 195–96
Bloating, 96
Blood-thinning
　drugs, 90
Blueberry muffins, 243
Blue cheese dressing, 218
Body fat, 66
Body weight, 9
Boiled potatoes, 167
Boneless chicken breast sautéed, 129
Braised lamb shanks, 122
Bran, 91
Bran muffins, 244
Bread, 8, 222
Brine, 61
Broccoli, steamed, 150
Broiled grapefruit, 186
Brown rice, 159
Café au lait, 232
Calcium, 4, 18
Calories, 3
Canned vegetables, 154
Carbohydrates, 2–3
Carrot and raisin salad, 207

265

Carrots, 151
Cereal, 8
Cheese, 194
Cheese quesadillas, 197
Cheese recipes
  cheese blintzes, 195–96
  cheese quesadillas, 197
  grilled cheese sandwiches, 225
  macaroni and cheese, 143
  quiche, 202
  stuffed shells, 146
Chef's salad, 208
Chemotherapeutic agents, 91
Chicken broth, 106
Chicken cutlets breaded, 130
Chicken fricassee, 131
Chicken grilled, 132
Chicken marinated, 133
Chicken parmigiana, 134
Chicken recipes
  boneless chicken breast sautéed, 129
  chicken cutlets breaded, 130
  chicken fricassee, 131
  chicken grilled, 132
  chicken marinated, 133
  chicken parmigiana, 134
  chicken/turkey sausage with onions, peppers, and mushrooms, 135
  tips for, 127–28
Chicken/turkey sausage with onions, peppers, and mushrooms, 135
Children
  diabetes in, 72
  foods to avoid for, 29
  guidelines for feeding, 25–27
  physical abilities of, 27–29
Chili, 116
Chinese-style fried rice, 160
Cholesterol
  controlling, 66, 78
  dietary fiber and, 78
  explanation of, 2, 67
  reducing intake of, 10, 68, 193
Cholesterol-lowering drugs, 91
Chronic conditions, 14
Cleaning up, 29
Clear liquid diets, 79–80
Clients, 22–25
Cobalamine, 17
Coffee, enriched ice, 234
Cole slaw, 209
Commercial thickeners, 82
Communication, age-appropriate, 23, 30

Complex carbohydrates, 2
Constipation, 99
Convenience foods, 45
Cooking guidelines, 55–56
Corn bread, 245
Creamsicle, 233
Creole fish, 139
Cross-contamination, 56
Cultural practices
  awareness of, 11, 12, 34–35
  changing, 34
  eating styles and, 33
  food choices and, 31–33

Dairy products, 8, 44, 194
Dates, food product, 55
Defrosting foods, 54
Dehydration, 99, 100
Department of Agriculture, U. S., 6
Department of Health and Human Services, U. S., 6
Diabetes
  explanation of, 71
  forms of, 72
  insulin shock and, 75
  risk factors for, 71–72
  signs and symptoms of, 72–73
Diabetic coma, 74–75
Diabetic diet
  guidelines for, 73–76
  importance of, 73
  when eating in restaurants, 74
Diarrhea, 99–100
Dietary fiber
  explanation of, 77–78
  intake of, 79, 83
  sources of, 78
Dietary Guidelines for Americans, 9–12
Dietary lipids, 66
Dietary supplements, 13–14. *See also* Supplements
Diets
  changes in, 34
  clear liquid, 79–80
  diabetic, 73–76
  dysphagia, 82
  fat- and cholesterol-restricted, 68–70, 193
  full liquid, 80–81
  low-lactose or lactose-free, 82–83
  low-residue or low-fiber, 79, 80
  mechanical soft, 81
  prescribed, 9

pureed, 81–82
sodium-restricted, 60–64
soft, 81
therapeutic, 11
Dry beans, 8
Dysphagia diet, 82

Eating practices, 33
Echinacea, 92
Edema, 96
Eggplant parmigiana, 142
Egg recipes
　blintzes, 195–96
　egg salad, 198
　french toast, 199
　omelet, 201
　quiche, 202
　strata, 203
Eggs
　Food Pyramid guidelines for, 8
　nutrients in, 193
　storage and handling of, 53, 193
Egg salad, 198
Egg substitutes, 193
Elderly people, 86–87
Endocrine system, 71
Energy, 66
English muffin pizza, 224
Enriched iced coffee, 234
Enteral nutrition, 100–101
Entree recipes
　beef, 113–120
　chicken and turkey, 127–136
　fish, 137–140
　lamb, 121–23
　meatless, 141–46
　pork, 124–26
Enzymes, 2
Essential fatty acids, 2

Fats
　explanation of, 2, 4, 66
　reducing intake of, 10, 65, 69, 70, 193
　sources of, 4, 66
　substitutes for, 69–70
　types of, 67
Fat-soluble vitamins, 16
Feeding
　assistive devices for, 23–24
　basic considerations for, 23
　children, 25–29
　cleaning up after, 29
　guidelines for, 29–30
　need for assistance with, 22
　overview of, 21
　planning for, 22–23
　safety factors related to, 24–25, 29
Fiber. *See* Dietary fiber
Fish
　Food Pyramid guidelines for, 8
　preparation of, 137
　storage and handling of, 51, 137
Fish recipes
　baked fish, 138
　creole fish, 139
　pan-fried fish, 140
　tips for, 137
Flatus, 97
Folacin, 17
Folic acid, 17
Food labels, 45, 46
Food poisoning, 49
Food Pyramid
　explanation of, 6–8
　guidelines for, 8–9
　use of, 10–12, 14
Foods. *See also specific foods*
　availability of specific, 32
　buying seasonal, 46–47
　convenience, 45
　cultural practices related to, 11, 12, 31–35
　dating of, 55
　defrosting, 54
　interactions between medication and, 85, 86, 89–93
　intolerances for specific, 12
　noting reactions to, 101–2
　to prevent or decrease, 99
　processed, 32
　sensible choices for, 10–11
Foods shopping
　guidelines for, 44, 47, 48
　making cost decisions during, 46–47
　planning for, 43–44
　reading labels when, 45, 46
　steps following, 47
　unit pricing and, 45
Food storage/handling
　cultural aspects of, 32
　dating food products and, 55
　defrosting and, 54
　freezer use and, 53
　guidelines for, 49, 52, 56, 57

Index **267**

Food storage/handling *(continued)*
  microwave use and, 53–54
  pantry use and, 54–55
  refrigerator use and, 50–51, 53
  safety issues related to, 50, 55–56
Freezer burn, 53
Freezer staples, 39
Freezer use, 53
French toast, 199
Fried rice Chinese style, 160
Frittata, 200
Fritters, 246
Frozen vegetables, 155
Fruit
  fiber in, 78, 183
  Food Pyramid guidelines for, 8
  guidelines for choosing, 183
  nutrients in, 183
  preparation of, 183–84
Fruit compote, 187
Fruit cubes, 188
Fruit freeze, 235
Fruit recipes
  baked apples, 185
  broiled grapefruit, 186
  cooked fruit compote, 187
  fruit cubes, 188
  glazed bananas, 189
  nectarine and cantaloupe smoothie, 190
  pureed fruit with whipped topping, 191
Fruity spread for graham crackers, 247
Full liquid diet, 80–81

Gas (flatus), 97
Gastrostomy, 101
Gestational diabetes, 72
Ginseng, 92
Glucose, 59
Grain recipes
  barley with mushrooms, 178
  grits casserole, 179
  quinoa, 180
  tabbouleh, 181
Grapefruit, broiled, 186
Grated zucchini, 152
Green beans sauté, 153
Grilled cheese sandwiches, 225
Grits casserole, 179

HDL (high-density lipoprotein), 67
Health care professionals, 2
Heart-related drugs, 91
Herbal supplements, 15, 88–92
Herbs
  explanation of, 15
  interactions between medication and, 89, 91–92
  in sodium-restricted diets, 63
  as staples, 39
Home fried potatoes, 168
Hormone replacement, 90
Hormones, 2
Hot apple cider, 236
Hydrogenated oils, 67
Hydrogenation, 2–3

Indian-style brown rice, 162
Infants, 28
Insoluble fiber, 78
Insulin, 71
Insulin shock, 75
Iodine, sources of, 4
Iron, 4, 18

Jejunostomy, 101

Kosher practices, 32, 61, 127

Lactose, 80
Lactose-free diets, 82–83
Lacto-vegetarians, 11
Lamb chops, 123
Lamb recipes
  braised lamb shanks, 122
  lamb chops, 123
  tips for, 121
LDL (low-density lipoprotein), 67
Lemon garlic mayonnaise, 219
Lentil soup, 107
Lentils with rice, 165
Licorice, 91
Lifecycle, 1
Lipids, 66
Low-fiber diet, 79, 80
Low-lactose diet, 82–83
Low-residue diet, 79, 80

Macaroni and cheese, 143
Magnesium, 18
Marinate, 56
Mashed potatoes, 169
Meals, 87
Meat
  cuts of, 113–14, 121
  Food Pyramid guidelines for, 8

guidelines for buying, 127
guidelines for cooking, 114, 124, 127–28
storage and handling of, 51
Meatless recipes
eggplant parmigiana, 142
English muffin pizza, 224
grilled cheese sandwiches, 225
macaroni and cheese, 143
pasta primavera, 144
quick tomato sauce, 145
roasted vegetable sandwiches, 226
stuffed shells, 146
tips for, 141
Meatloaf, 117
Meat recipes
beef, 113–120
chicken and turkey, 127–136
lamb, 121–23
pork, 124–26
Mechanical soft diet, 81
Medication
for diabetes, 74–76
interactions between alcohol and, 92
interactions between food and, 85, 86, 89–93
interactions between herbs and, 89, 91–92
interactions between supplements and, 15
reactions to, 93
storage of, 88
understanding labels for, 88
Mexican-style rice, 163
Micronutrients, 3
Microorganisms, 50
Microwave ovens, 53–54, 56
Milligrams, 60
Minerals, 3–4, 18
Minestrone soup, 108
Moderation, 7, 12
Monounsaturated fats, 67
Mouth soreness, 97, 98
Mushrooms with barley, 178

Nasogastric feeding, 101
National Cholesterol Education Program, 68
Nausea, 98–99
Nectarine and cantalope smoothie, 190
Niacin, 5, 16

Nutrients, 1–3
Nuts, 8

Oatmeal, 78, 91
Olestra (Olean), 69–70
Omelet, 201
Ovo-vegetarians, 11
Oxidation, 15

Pan-fried fish, 140
Pantothenic acid, 17
Pantries, 54–55
Pantry staples, 40
Pasta
with beans, 173
with butter, 174
with garlic and oil, 175
guidelines for, 8, 157
with herbs and cheese, 176
primavera, 144
with quick tomato sauce, 177
stuffed shells, 146
Pasteurized dairy products, 44
Peas, 78
Pepper steak, 118
Peristalsis, 79
Permeable wrappings, 53
Phosphorus, 4, 18
Physical abilities, 27–29
Physical activity, 9
Phytochemicals, 15
Pizza English muffin, 224
Polyunsaturated fats, 67
Pork, 124
Pork medallions, 125
Pork stir-fry, 126
Portions, 26, 27
Potassium, 18
Potatoes
baked, 166
boiled, 167
croquettes, 170
home fried, 168
mashed, 169
roasted, 172
rosemary garlic sweet, 171
Potato salad, 210
Pot roast, 119
Poultry
Food Pyramid guidelines for, 8
preparation of, 127–28
recipes for, 127–136
storage and handling of, 51, 127

Pregnancy, 60, 72
Prescribed diets, 9
Processed foods, 32
Protein
 cost issues when buying foods high in, 47
 explanation of, 2
 sources of, 3
Psyllium, 78
Pureed diets, 81–82
Pureed fruit with whipped topping, 191
Pyridoxine, 17

Quiche, 202
Quick tomato sauce, 145
Quinoa, 180

Raisin oatmeal bars, 248
Recipes
 beef, 115–120
 beverage, 231–39
 cheese, 143, 195–97, 202, 225
 egg, 195–96, 198, 199, 201–3
 fish, 138–140
 fruit, 185–191
 grain, 178–181
 lamb, 122–23
 meatless, 142–46
 pasta, 146, 173–77
 pork, 125–26
 potato, 166–172
 poultry, 129–136
 rice, 159–165
 salad, 207–215
 salad dressing, 216–19
 sandwich, 224–27
 snack, 242–49
 soup, 103–112
 vegetable side-dish, 149–155
Reference diet, 45
Refrigerator staples, 38
Refrigerator use, 50–51, 53
Religious practices, 32
Restaurants, 74
Riboflavin, 5, 17
Rice, 8, 157
Rice and beans, 161
Rice and vegetable salad, 211
Rice Indian style, 162
Rice Mexican style, 163
Rice pilaf, 164
Rice pudding, 249

Rice recipes
 brown rice, 159
 fried rice Chinese style, 160
 rice and beans, 161
 rice Indian style, 162
 rice Mexican style, 163
 rice pilaf, 164
 rice with lentils, 165
 tips for, 157
Rice with lentils, 165
Roasted potatoes, 172
Roasted vegetable sandwiches, 226
Rosemary garlic sweet potatoes, 171

Safety issues
 for eating sandwiches, 223
 for feeding clients, 24–25, 29
 for food storage and handling, 50, 55–56
Salad dressings
 balsamic vinaigrette, 216
 basic lemon, 217
 blue cheese, 218
 lemon garlic mayonnaise, 219
 tips for, 205–206
Salad recipes
 carrot and raisin salad, 207
 chef's salad, 208
 cole slaw, 209
 potato salad, 210
 rice and vegetable salad, 211
 spinach salad, 212
 three-bean salad, 213
 tuna fish salad, 214
 vegetable salad, 215
Salads, 205–6
Salt, 10. *See also* Sodium
Sandwiches
 accompaniments for, 223
 breads for, 222
 explanation of, 221
 fillings for, 222
Sandwich recipes
 English muffin pizza, 224
 grilled cheese sandwiches, 225
 roasted vegetable sandwiches, 226
 turkey and cheese roll-up, 227
Saturated fats, 2, 10, 67
Semi-vegetarians, 11
Simple carbohydrates, 2
Sloppy joes, 120
Snack recipes
 apple crisp, 242
 blueberry muffins, 243

bran muffins, 244
corn bread, 245
fritters, 246
fruity spread for graham crackers, 247
raisin oatmeal bars, 248
rice pudding, 249
Snacks, 241
Sodium
 foods high in, 62
 reducing intake of, 10
 requirements for, 59, 60
Sodium-restricted diets
 effects of, 61
 guidelines for, 60–61, 63, 64
 tips for, 61–62
 using herbs and spices in, 63
Soft diet, 81
Soluble fiber, 78
Sore throat, 97, 98
Soup recipes
 bean, 105
 braised lamb shanks, 122
 chicken broth, 106
 lentil, 107
 minestrone, 108
 split pea, 109
 tips for, 103
 tomato, 110
 turkey vegetable, 111
 vegetable, 112
Spices, 39, 63
Spinach salad, 212
Split pea soup, 109
Staples
 explanation of, 37–38
 freezer, 39
 herbs and spices as, 39
 making decisions about, 41
 pantry, 40
 refrigerator, 38
Strata, 203
Strawberry milk smoothie, 237
Stuffed shells, 146
Sugar, 10
Supplements
 dietary, 13–14
 explanation of, 1–2, 13
 guidelines for, 19
 herbal and antioxidant, 15
 interactions between medication and, 15
 supervision of, 18–19

 support for clients taking, 14–15
 vitamin and mineral, 16–18
Sweet potatoes, 171
Synthesized, 2

Tabbouleh, 181
Thawing, 54
Therapeutic diets, 11
Thiamine, 5, 16
Three-bean salad, 213
Throat, sore, 97, 98
Toddlers, 28
Tomato sauce, 145
Tomato soup, 110
Total parenteral nutrition (TPN), 101
Tuna fish salad, 214
Turkey and cheese roll-up, 227
Turkey burgers, 136
Turkey sausage with onions, peppers, and mushrooms, 135
Turkey vegetable soup, 111

Unaffected side, 24
Unit pricing, 45
Unsaturated fats, 2

Vanilla milkshake, 238
Vegans, 11
Vegetables
 canned, 155
 Food Pyramid guidelines for, 8
 frozen, 155
 tips for cooking, 147–48
Vegetable salad, 215
Vegetable side-dish recipes
 baked acorn squash, 149
 with canned vegetables, 154
 carrots, 151
 frozen vegetables, 155
 grated zucchini, 152
 green beans sauté, 153
 potato, 166–172
 steamed broccoli, 150
 tips for, 147–48
Vegetable soup, 112
Vegetarian recipes
 eggplant parmigiana, 142
 English muffin pizza, 224
 grilled cheese sandwiches, 225
 macaroni and cheese, 143
 pasta primavera, 144
 quick tomato sauce, 145
 roasted vegetable sandwiches, 226

Index **271**

Vegetarian recipes *(continued)*
  stuffed shells, 146
  tips for, 141
Vegetarians, 11
Vitamin A, 5, 15, 16
Vitamin B_1, 5, 16
Vitamin B_2, 5, 17
Vitamin B_3, 16
Vitamin B_6, 17
Vitamin B_{12}, 5, 17
Vitamin B complex, 5
Vitamin C, 6, 15, 17
Vitamin D, 6, 17
Vitamin E, 15, 17
Vitamin K, 18

Vitamins
  antioxidant, 15
  explanation of, 3, 16
  fat-soluble, 16
  sources of, 5–6, 15–18
  water-soluble, 16
VLDL (very low-density lipoprotein), 67
Vomiting, 98–99

Water, 6
Water-soluble vitamins, 16

Yogurt smoothie, 239